POLYCYSTIC OVARY SYNDROME

Edited by **Srabani Mukherjee**

Polycystic Ovary Syndrome
Edited by Srabani Mukherjee

Published by InTech

Janeza Trdine 9, 51000 Rijeka, Croatia

Publishing Process Manager Molly Kaliman

Technical Editor Teodora Smiljanic

Cover Designer InTech Design Team

Additional hard copies can be obtained from orders@intechopen.com

Polycystic Ovary Syndrome, Edited by Srabani Mukherjee
p. cm.
ISBN 978-953-51-0094-2

For EU product safety concerns:
IN TECH d.o.o., Prolaz Marije Krucifikse Kozulić 3, 51000 Rijeka, Croatia,
info@intechopen.com or visit our website at intechopen.com.

Meet the editor

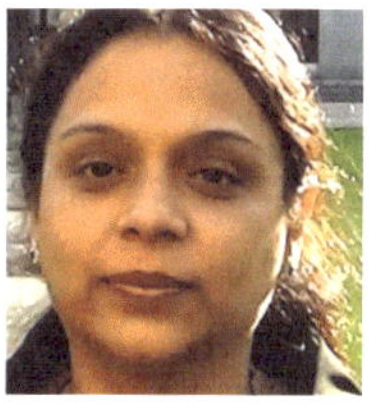

Dr Mukherjee is at present an assistant director at the National Institute for Research in Reproductive Health (NIRRH) in Mumbai, a premier research institution under the purview of the Indian Council of Medical Research and the Ministry of Health. She has earned her Bachelor of Science and her Masters degree in Physiology from the University of Calcutta. She has received her doctorate in Biochemistry from the Indian Institute of Chemical Biology. Subsequently she has been affiliated as a research associate with the Indian Institute of Technology, Mumbai and the P.D. Hinduja National Hospital and Research Centre. She received Post-doctoral training at University of Texas Health Science Centre at San Antonio, USA. She is a Fellow in "Frontiers in Reproduction Marine Biological Laboratory" at MBL, Woods Hole, USA. She is a member of Indian Society for Study of Reproduction and Fertility (ISSRF) and been awarded several research grants to carry out her research work. She has extensive hands-on expertise in a variety of current molecular biology techniques, protein and cell culture practices. Her position as head of the flow cytometry facility at NIRRH and her attendance at various trainings has made her highly experienced in this technique. Dr Mukherjee has delivered many talks at various conferences and authored several publications in the field of molecular biology and reproduction. She has been pursuing active research over the last twenty years and her keen interests currently lie in infertility studies with focus on the Polycystic Ovary Syndrome, a common endocrinopathy in females of reproductive age. She is presently working towards understanding the pathophysiology of Polycystic Ovary Syndrome (PCOS) by genetic profiling and proteomics studies.

Contents

Preface

"The beginning of knowledge is the discovery of something we do not understand."
Frank Herbert (1920-1986)

Polycystic Ovary Syndrome (PCOS) is a common heterogenous disorder in women of reproductive age. It is a leading cause of anovulatory infertility all over the world. Having an early onset during pre-pubertal years, it has been associated with many reproductive complications. Over the years there has been a paradigm shift in thought; it is no longer just a gynecological concern but has a strong metabolic component too. Women with PCOS have a markedly increased risk of developing central obesity, Type 2 Diabetes and cardiovascular diseases. Research in this field has been progressing at an incredible rate, however even with staggering data available, researchers have not been able to fully understand this endocrine enigma. Questions regarding its pathophysiology and its possible long-term reproductive and metabolic outcomes are being tackled by rigorous research, but no definite conclusions have been reached yet. The focus in this book is drawn towards understanding the clinical and metabolic manifestations, as well as the impact that they have on the psychosocial well-being in women with PCOS. Some therapeutic options such as the use of insulin sensitizing agents and ovulation inducers to improve fertility, as well as impact of lifestyle and dietary modifications to reduce obesity and its associated consequences, have been highlighted in this text. Analysis of this ongoing research has incited the search for alternative and improved treatments to alleviate these health concerns with great zeal. This book aims to offer fellow researchers a comprehensive overview of the current knowledge of the developments in this expanding field.

Srabani Mukherjee
Department of Molecular Endocrinology,
National Institute for Research in Reproductive Health (ICMR), Mumbai,
India

1

Management of Women with Clomifene Citrate Resistant Polycystic Ovary Syndrome – An Evidence Based Approach

Hatem Abu Hashim
Department of Obstetrics & Gynecology, Faculty of Medicine, Mansoura University, Mansoura, Egypt

1. Introduction

World Health Organisation (WHO) type II anovulation is defined as normogonadotrophic normoestrogenic anovulation and occurs in approximately 85% of anovulatory patients. Polycystic ovary syndrome (PCOS) is the most common form of WHO type II anovulatory infertility and is associated with hyperandrogenemia (1,2). Moreover, PCOS is the most common endocrine abnormality in reproductive age women. The prevalence of PCOS is traditionally estimated at 4% to 8% from studies performed in Greece, Spain and the USA (3-6). The prevalence of PCOS has increased with the use of different diagnostic criteria and has recently been shown to be 11.9 ± 2.4% -17.8 ± 2.8 in the first community-based prevalence study based on the current Rotterdam diagnostic criteria compared with 10.2 ± 2.2% -12.0 ± 2.4% and 8.7 ± 2.0% using National Institutes of Health criteria and Androgen Excess Society recommendations respectively (7). Importantly, 70% of women in this recent study were undiagnosed (7).

Clomiphene citrate (CC) is still holding its place as the first-line therapy for ovulation induction in these patients (2,8,9). CC contains an unequal mixture of two isomers as their citrate salts, enclomiphene and zuclomiphene. Zuclomiphene is much the more potent of the two for induction of ovulation, accounts for 38% of the total drug content of one tablet and has a much longer half-life than enclomiphene, being detectable in plasma 1 month following its administration (10). CC is capable of inducing a discharge of FSH from the anterior pituitary and this is often enough to reset the cycle of events leading to ovulation into motion. This is achieved indirectly, through the action of CC, a non-steroidal compound closely resembling an estrogen, in blocking hypothalamic estrogen receptors, signalling a lack of circulating estrogen to the hypothalamus and inducing a change in the pattern of pulsatile release of GnRH(10). Standard practice is to administer CC for 5 days from the second or third day of the menstrual cycle, starting with 50mg/day and increasing to 250mg/day (10). However managed care studies have shown that the most effective dosage is 100–150mg/day and over 75% of ovulations occur within these dosages (11). After six to nine cycles of treatment with CC cumulative pregnancy rates reach 70–75% (11). Life table analysis of the most reliable studies indicated a conception rate up to 22% per cycle in women ovulating on CC (8). In a large randomized trial, Legro et al., 2007 (12) compared the effects of CC, metformin and combination therapy in 626 infertile women with PCOS. They reported an ovulation and clinical pregnancy rates per woman of 75.1% and 23.9% respectively, after CC treatment up to 150mg/day.

Clomiphene resistance defined as failure to ovulate after receiving 150 mg of CC daily for 5 days per cycle, for at least three cycles, is common and occurs in approximately 15 to 40% in women with PCOS (2, 13). Insulin resistance, hyperandrogenemia, and obesity represent the major factors involved in CC resistance; avert the ovaries from responding to raised endogenous FSH levels following CC therapy (14-16). Moreover, a genetic predisposition was suggested (17).

The purpose of this chapter is to review the evidence based treatment strategies for ovulation induction in anovulatory PCOS patients with known CC resistance, both the traditional and new ones. The traditional options include gonadotrophins and surgery (laparoscopic ovarian drilling). New strategies as insulin-sensitizing drugs, aromatase Inhibitors, oral contraceptives, dexamethasone, N-acetyl-cysteine…etc. Moreover, optimizing the body mass index (BMI) firstly before commencing therapy is an important issue to improve the treatment outcome in obese anovulatory women with PCOS. In vitro fertilization (IVF) is the recommended line of treatment after failure of these strategies; however, it is outside the scope of this chapter. Finally an algorithm will be provided to facilitate management of this important clinical issue.

2. Weight loss and lifestyle modifications

Obesity is strongly associated with PCOS and may be present in up to 50% of cases (18-22). Obese women with PCOS are more likely than thin women with PCOS to suffer from anovulation (18). This effect on ovulation may be secondary to insulin resistance, which in turn results in hyperinsulinemia and stimulation of excess androgen production from the ovaries (22). Lifestyle modification is the first line treatment in an evidence based approach for the management of the majority of PCOS women who are overweight (8,9,13, 23-25). The NICE, 2004 (13) recommended weight loss for anovulatory PCOS women who have a BMI > 29 kg/m2 before starting ovulation induction therapy. In these women, weight loss of even 5% to 10% of body weight often restores ovulatory cycles (9, 19, 21). Studies also showed that overweight women are less likely to respond to pharmacologic ovulation induction methods. In a cohort of 270 women, with PCOS who received either CC or gonadotrophins for ovulation induction, almost 80% with a BMI of 18–24 kg/m2 ovulated at 6 months compared with only 12% of women with a BMI≥35 kg/m2 (18). Moreover, overweight women require higher doses of CC and gonadotrophins (19).

The current recommendation is to reduce weight gradually to increase the chances of maintaining the weight loss (9). Preferential diet composition has been evaluated in 2 small studies (26, 27). These studies compared a high carbohydrate (55%), low protein (15%) hypocaloric diet with a low carbohydrate (40%), high protein (30%) hypocaloric diet and found similar weight loss and decrease in circulating androgen and insulin levels. Routine exercise is also very important in the reproductive health of PCOS women. Exercise increases insulin sensitivity and helps achieve and maintain weight loss (9, 25). Incorporating simple moderate physical activity including structured exercise (at least 30 min/ day) and incidental exercise increases weight loss and improves clinical outcomes in PCOS, compared to diet alone (28). Also, a recent study reported that a 6-week intervention of structured exercise training and a hypocaloric diet was effective in increasing the probability of ovulation under CC treatment in overweight and obese CC-resistant PCOS patients (29). Other lifestyle factors such as excessive caffeine intake, alcohol consumption, and smoking should also be addressed (13,20).

Otta et al., 2010 (30) in a randomized, double-blind, and placebo control trial compared lifestyle modification and 1500 mg of metformin or placebo for 4 months in 30 women with insulin resistance PCOS. They reported that metformin has an additive effect to diet and exercise to improve parameters of hyperandrogenism and insulin resistance. However, a small decrease in body weight through lifestyle changes could be enough to improve menstrual cycles in these women. Karimzadeh & Javedani, 2010 (31)in another randomized double-blind study compared lifestyle modification with medical treatment plans such as CC, metformin, and CC with metformin in 343 overweight infertile women with PCOS. They showed that metformin or metformin with CC does not cause a significant weight loss or an improvement in the endocrine status of PCOS women. However, lifestyle modification to reduce waist circumference and body weight could improve their menstrual cycles, hormonal status and was an effective treatment for ovulation induction in those patients with an ovulation and pregnancy rates of 66.6% and 20% respectively.

In morbidly obese women, the PCOS phenotype appears to be very frequent (32). Importantly, this disorder has been found to improve markedly after sustained weight loss following bariatric surgery (33). Anti-obesity pharmacological agents have been used in obese women with PCOS. Both orlistat, which blocks intestinal absorption of fat (34), and sibutramine, an appetite suppressant (35), have displayed a weight loss-independent effect on androgens and insulin resistance. It should be noted that these treatments should not be considered as first-line therapy for obesity in women with PCOS (8).

3. Gonadotrophins

Ovulation induction for women with anovulatory PCOS using gonadotrophin therapy is based on the physiological concept that initiation and maintenance of follicle growth may be achieved by a transient increase in FSH above a threshold dose for sufficient duration to generate a limited number of developing follicles (8). Traditionally, Ovulation induction with gonadotrophins has been used as a second line treatment for CC-resistant PCOS women, however it is expensive, requires extensive monitoring and associated with significantly increased risk for ovarian hyperstimulation syndrome (OHSS) and multiple pregnancy (8, 9, 13, 36-38). Furthermore, a significant and consistent relationship between PCOS and OHSS was reported in a systematic review (39). The high sensitivity of the PCOS to gonadotrophic stimulation is probably related to the fact that they contain twice the number of available follicle-stimulating hormone (FSH)-sensitive antral follicles in their cohort than the normal ovary (40). A meta-analysis concluded that the outcomes of treatment achieved with hMG and with FSH alone in infertile patients with PCOS were similar except for a reduction in the risk of OHSS with the urinary FSH (uFSH) (41). A low-dose, step-up gonadotrophin therapy should be preferred to the now outdated conventional protocol for patients with PCOS and the strong justification seems to be; the achievement of high rate of mono-follicular development which is ~69% (54–88%) (36,42) with nearly complete elimination of OHSS (0–2.4%) and a multiple pregnancy rate of ~6% (36,43). The recommended approach is to begin with a low dose of gonadotrophin, typically 37.5- 75

IU/day, increasing after 7 days or more if no follicle >10 mm has yet emerged, in small increments, at intervals, until evidence of progressive follicular development is observed. The maximum required daily dose of FSH/hMG seldom exceeds 225 IU/day (38, 44). There is no evidence of a difference between recombinant FSH (rFSH) and uFSH for ovulation induction in CC- resistant PCOS women (45,46). In addition, a randomised trial (RCT) of highly purified uFSH (HP-uFSH) versus rFSH found that the former was non-inferior compared with the latter with respect to ovulation rate (85.2% versus 90.9%) in anovulatory WHO Group II women who failed to ovulate or conceive on CC (47) .

4. Laparoscopic Ovarian Diathermy (LOD)

Laparoscopic ovarian diathermy (LOD) is currently accepted as a successful second line treatment for ovulation induction in CC-resistant PCOS being as effective as gonadotrophin treatment and is not associated with an increased risk of multiple pregnancy or OHSS (8, 9,13, 48-51). Bayram et al., 2004 (50) in a RCT compared LOD with rFSH in 168 CC-resistant PCOS women. They reported an ovulation rate of 70% and 69% per cycle and pregnancy and live-birth rates 37%, 75% and 34%, 60% of patients respectively following LOD and FSH therapy. In patients remaining anovulatory 8 weeks after LOD or those who subsequently became anovulatory, adjuvant therapy with CC or gonadotrophins was required to achieve equivalent pregnancy and live-birth rates (50). A Cochrane review found no difference in the rates of miscarriage, ongoing pregnancy or live birth between LOD and gonadotrophins. Multiple pregnancy rates were significantly lower with LOD than with gonadotrophins (1% versus 16%; OR 0.13, 95% CI 0.03 to 0.52) (49). A recent study concluded that LOD for women with CC-resistant PCOS is as effective as ovulation induction with rFSH treatment in terms of live births, but reduces the need for ovulation induction or ART in a significantly higher proportion of women and increases the chance for a second child (52).

The main shortcomings of LOD are the need for general anesthesia and the risk of postoperative adhesions (53, 54). The claim that it might affect the ovarian reserve is not more than a theoretical concern since a recent report concluded that LOD, when applied properly, does not seem to compromise the ovarian reserve in PCOS women (55). Moreover, an economic evaluation has shown that the cost of a live birth after LOD is approximately one-third lower than the equivalent cost of gonadotrophin treatment (56). The most commonly used energy for LOD is electrocautery. It has been reported that the clinical and endocrine response to LOD is governed by a dose response relationship. Four punctures per ovary using a power setting of 30 W applied for 5s per puncture (i.e. 600 J per ovary) are sufficient to produce an optimal response (67% spontaneous ovulation rate and 67% conception rate). Reducing the thermal energy below that level reduces the chances of spontaneous ovulation and conception (57). Also, different studies argued for unilateral LOD being equally efficacious as bilateral drilling in inducing ovulation and achieving pregnancy in CC resistant PCOS patients and may be regarded as a suitable option with the potential advantage of decreasing the chances of adhesion formation (58-60).

Although it remains unclear as to how LOD induces ovulation, a potential mechanism is that LOD drains the ovarian follicles containing a high concentration of androgens and inhibin, which causes the reduction of blood androgens and blood inhibin resulting in an increase of FSH and recovery of the ovulation function (51,53, 61,62). Surgery may also provoke an increased blood flow to the ovary, allowing increased delivery of gonadotrophins (53, 62). Women with marked obesity (BMI >35 kg/m2), marked hyperandrogenism (serum testosterone concentration >4.5 nmol/l, free androgen index (FAI) >15) and/or long duration of infertility (>3 years) seem to be poor responders to LOD. On the other hand, high LH levels >10 IU/l in LOD responders appear to predict higher probability of pregnancy (63). van Wely et al., 2005 (64) reported that women who had an age at menarche < 13years, an LH/FSH ratio < 2 and a glucose level < 4.5 mmol/l, were more likely to remain anovulatory following LOD.

Restoration of consecutive spontaneous ovulations after LOD in some CC-resistant PCOS patients is one of the most important advantages of this approach (65). Another potential advantage is the increased responsiveness of the ovary to oral ovulation induction agents following the procedure. In a recent study, we evaluated whether LOD in CC-resistant PCOS patients led to the restoration of CC-sensitivity. LOD was performed in 234 CC-resistant PCOS patients. In 150 patients ovulation occurred. The remaining 84 aonvulatory patients were again treated with CC. Ovulation occurred in 30 /84 patients (35.7%), meanwhile, pregnancy occurred in 13/ 84 patients (15.5%). Hyperandrogenism and insulin resistance were negative predictors (66).

5. Insulin-sensitizing drugs

Approximately 50%-70% of all women with PCOS have some degree of insulin resistance (67). Hyperinsulinemia probably contributes to the hyperandrogenism which is responsible for the signs and symptoms of PCOS (67). Metformin, a biguanide, is now the most widely insulin sensitizer used for ovulation induction in women with PCOS. In these women, it appears to affect ovarian function in a dual mode, through the alleviation of insulin excess acting upon the ovary and through direct ovarian effects. Being an insulin sensitizer, it reduces insulin secretion and, consequently, lowers circulating total and free androgen levels with a resulting improvement of the clinical sequelae of hyperandrogenism. Importantly, it also seems to have a direct action on ovarian theca cells to decrease androgen production (68). A recent meta-analysis of RCTs showd no significant difference in effectiveness of metformin versus CC as a first-line treatment for ovulation induction in non-obese women with anovulatory PCOS (69). Also a recent Cochrane review reported that metformin is still of benefit in improving clinical pregnancy and ovulation rates. However, there is no evidence that it improves live birth rates whether it is used alone or in combination with CC, or when compared with CC. Therefore, the use of metformin as a first-line treatment in improving reproductive outcomes in women with PCOS appears to be limited (70).

Many investigators have demonstrated an improvement in insulin sensitivity and a significant decrease in serum insulin and free testosterone levels after long term treatment with metformin for 5–8 weeks (71-73). Creanga et al., 2008 (74) in a meta-analysis, confirmed that metformin in combination with CC increased the likelihood of ovulation [OR 4.39, 95% CI 1.94–9.96, number - needed- to-treat (NNT) 3.7] and pregnancy (OR 2.67, 95% CI 1.45–4.94, NNT 4.6) in comparison with CC alone, especially in CC-resistant and obese PCOS patients. Actually, different mechanisms explaining why metformin therapy would facilitate ovulation induction by CC in CC- resistant PCOS patients have been proposed entailing; an intrinsic alteration of follicle steroidogenesis through the IGF-I pathway in granulosa cells (73); direct inhibition of androgen production in ovarian thecal cells (75); reduction in the adrenal steroidogenesis response to ACTH (76) and recently its central action on the pituitary gland with an LH lowering and prolactin effects in the PCOS women (77). There are unpleasant gastrointestinal side effects including nausea, vomiting, bloating, cramps and diarrhoea. Rare complication includes lactic acidosis. Metformin has been used in increasing doses from 500 to 1500 mg daily for the induction of ovulation in women with PCOS (9).

Recently, the efficacy of the combination of metformin and CC versus other traditional options including gonadotrophins and LOD for treatment of CC-resistant infertile PCOS patients has been reported. Two RCTs compared the combination of metformin and CC with LOD, showing that both are effective approaches to treat CC- resistant infertile PCOS patients (78, 79). In fifty primary infertile patients with CC- resistant PCOS, Palombo et al., 2010 (78) found no significant difference between the 2 groups in pregnancy and live-birth rates per cycle (13.1% vs.16.3% and 11.2% vs. 14.1% respectively). However, the ovulation rate per cycle was significantly lower in LOD group than in Metformin/CC group (56.5% vs. 72.0%). On the other hand, in a well designed adequately powered RCT comprised of 282 anovulatory women with CC-resistant PCOS, we reported no significant difference between the 2 groups in ovulation and pregnancy rates per cycle (67% vs. 68.2% and 15.4% vs. 17% respectively). However, a significant difference regarding midcycle endometrial thickness was found (9.2 ± 1.2 mm vs. 7.6 ± 1.1 mm, in Metformin/CC and LOD groups respectively) (79). George et al., 2003 (80) in a small trial of limited power compared sequential treatment of metformin and CC with conventional hMG protocol in 60 CC-resistant PCOS patients. In this trial, metformin alone was given as a single pretreatment for 6 months, followed by ovulation induction with CC. There was no significant difference in pregnancy rates between the two groups (16.7 vs. 23.3%). However, in the metformin group, significant improvements in menstrual function and ovulation rate of 46.7% with a significant decrease in fasting insulin levels were reported. The ovulation rate in hMG group was 43.3%, with a high drop-out rate. Recently, in a well designed adequately powered RCT we compared the effects of combined metformin–CC with HP-uFSH using low-dose, step-up regimen for three cycles in 153 anovulatory women with CC-resistant PCOS (81). Actually, combined metformin-CC therapy was not expected to be more effective than gonadotrophins, however, it did result in modest ovulation and pregnancy rates. Ovulation and pregnancy rates per cycle were 62% vs. 83.8% and 11.2% vs. 21.5% in combined metformin- CC group and HP-uFSH groups respectively. HP-uFSH administration had good results, but, the low-dose, step-up regimen requires extensive monitoring and expertise, and has high costs. Accordingly, it is logical to offer combined metformin- CC therapy first in the step-wise treatment protocol for CC-resistant PCOS patients before resorting to more expensive alternatives especially in developing communities where economic aspects of therapy are important (81).

The safety of metformin has sparked a heated debate. Recent evidence that metformin is probably safe during the first trimester of pregnancy and beyond is accumulating (82-85). Moreover, a recent meta-analysis found no effect of pregestational metformin administration on abortion risk in PCOS patients (86). Other insulin sensitizers from the thiazolidenediones family, namely rosiglitazone, have been used effectively in CC-resistant PCOS patients. In a RCT, the combination of rosiglitazone and CC was reported to be more effective than metformin and CC in terms of ovulation rate (64.3 vs. 36.4%, respectively); whereas no statistical significance was observed in pregnancy rate (50 vs. 38.5%) (87). Also, a recent RCT reported no significant difference between combined treatment with rosiglitazone and CC vs. LOD in 43 CC-resistant PCOS patients in terms of biochemical response, ovulation rate (80.8 vs. 81.5%) and pregnancy rate (50 vs. 42.8%) (88). A retrospective analysis investigated various clinical, biochemical, and ultrasonographic factors that determine clinical response to rosiglitazone as a first-line therapy in a series of PCOS women with newly diagnosed CC-resistance. It showed that marked obesity, marked hyperandrogenism, and long duration of infertility were predictors of resistance to rosiglitazone therapy (89).

6. Third-generation aromatase inhibitors

Third-generation aromatase inhibitors (anastrozole, letrozole, exemestane) are approved adjuvants for treatment of estrogen-receptor–positive breast cancer (90) that were first used in ovulation induction in anovulatory women in 2001 (91). Evidence suggests that nonsteroidal aromatase inhibitors (AIs), specifically letrozole and anastrozole, have ovulation-inducing effects by inhibiting androgen-to-estrogen conversion. Centrally, this effect releases the hypothalamic/pituitary axis from estrogenic negative feedback, increases gonadotrophin secretion, and results in stimulation of ovarian follicle maturity. Moreover, peripherally, AIs may increase follicular sensitivity to FSH (92). AIs have relatively short half-lives (~2 days) compared with CC (~2 weeks) so estrogen target tissues (e.g., endometrium and cervix) are spared adverse effects. Because of these mechanisms, it was postulated that AIs may have superior ovulation induction properties in terms of follicular growth and endometrium development, which is important for embryo implantation (92).

Recent studies showed that letrozole has better ovulation and pregnancy rates in comparison to CC and placebo in patients with CC- resistant PCOS (93-96). There are 2 prospective studies in the literature comparing the two commercially available third generation AIs, letrozole and anastrozole in CC-resistant infertile women with PCOS. Al-Omari et al., 2004 (97) studied 40 cases who were considered CC- resistant if failed ovulation after 200 mg CC daily for 5 days or were ovulatory with an endometrium thickness less than 5 mm. Ovulation and pregnancy rates per cycle were significantly higher with letrozole compared with anastrozole (84.4% vs. 60% and 18.8% vs. 9.7%, respectively). Endometrium thickness was significantly greater for letrozole compared with anastrozole (8.16 ± 1.32 vs. 6.53 ± 1.55 mm). Multiple pregnancies did not occur. In this small trial, PCOS diagnostic criteria were not stated. Additionally, the dose of CC used to define resistance was very high, possibly suggesting an extremely refractory population. Importantly, a larger RCT compared the efficacy of letrozole and anastrozole in 220 CC–resistant women with PCOS diagnosed with Rotterdam criteria. More growing and mature follicles and greater endometrial thickness in patients receiving anastrozole were demonstrated; however, no significant advantage for anastrozole over letrozole with regard to ovulation, pregnancy or miscarriage rates was observed (63.4 vs.62% and 15.1vs. 12.2% and 9.5vs. 11.1% respectively). Two twin pregnancies occurred with letrozole, while none occurred with anastrozole (98). In the above mentioned 2 studies, a short course (5 days) of letrozole was used. However, a long letrozole protocol (10 days) was also proposed, with proved advantages in terms of more mature follicles and subsequently more pregnancies (99).

One small trial of limited power compared combined metformin–letrozole vs. metformin–CC in 60 CC-resistant PCOS patients reported that combined metformin–letrozole was associated with significantly more endometrial thickness, E2 levels and full-term pregnancy rate. However, no statistically significant difference was found between the two groups as regards the mean number of mature follicles, ovulation and pregnancy rates. The authors admitted that combined metformin- letrozole is better than letrozole alone, particularly in overweight women and asked for further studies to confirm their hypothesis (100). Recently, in a well designed adequately powered RCT, we compared the effects of letrozole monotherapy (2.5 mg daily for 5 days from D3-7 of the cycle) with combined metformin-CC in 250 anovulatory women (582 cycles) with CC resistant PCOS. Our findings suggested that letrozole monotherapy and combined metformin-CC were equally effective for inducing ovulation and achieving pregnancy in patients with CC-resistant PCOS (64.9% vs.69.6% and 14.7% vs. 14.4% respectively). The total number of follicles was significantly more in the combined metformin-CC group (4.4 ± 0.4 vs. 6.8 ± 0.3). A non significant increase in endometrial thickness on the day of hCG administration was observed in the letrozole group (9.5 ± 0.2 mm vs. 9.1 ± 0.1 mm). Since letrozole was well tolerated, it is considered as an acceptable alternative if CC-resistant PCOS patients cannot tolerate long-term metformin pretreatment (101).

More recently, the efficacy of the AIs vs. other traditional options including gonadotrophins and LOD for treatment of CC-resistant infertile PCOS patients has been reported. 2 RCTs compared the effect of letrozole (2.5mg and 5 mg respectively from day 3 to day 7 of menses for 6 consecutive cycles) with LOD for ovulation induction in CC resistant women with PCOS. Both trials reported that letrozole and LOD are equally effective for inducing ovulation and achieving pregnancy in these patients. Moreover, women in the letrozole group had a significantly thicker endometrium than those in the LOD group. In view of the invasiveness and cost of surgery, it seems plausible that letrozole therapy should be tried first for most of those women before shifting to LOD (102,103). A recent large randomized trial by Ganesh et al., 2009 (104) compared the efficacy of letrozole with that of rFSH and CC/rFSH for ovarian stimulation in IUI cycles in 1387 PCOS women after CC failure. They reported an ovulation rate of 79.30% in letrozole group vs. 56.95% and 89.89% in other groups respectively and pregnancy rate of 23.39% in letrozole group vs. 14.35% and 17.92% in other groups respectively. However, they included not only CC-resistant PCOS patients but also those who failed to conceive with100 mg/day CC for 6 cycles despite ovulating and those who showed poor endometrial development i.e. endometrial thickness < 7 mm on the day of hCG administration.

Letrozole was evaluated in 44 women with CC-resistant PCOS and both responders and nonresponders were characterized. PCOS was diagnosed by Rotterdam criteria; CC-resistance was defined as failure to ovulate after 6 cycles of 150 mg CC /day for 5 days. Whereas response to CC is less likely with elevated BMI, amenorrhea, and increased age, significant differences between letrozole responders and nonresponders were not noted for any evaluated measure. This apparent lack of predictive factors for letrozole suggests utility in CC-resistant patients since its efficacy is not limited to specific patient characteristics (105). The safety of letrozole has elaborated a vivid discussion. Preliminary data by Biljan et al., 2005 (106) suggested an increased risk of congenital anomalies in letrozole treated babies, whereas recent data from retrospective and prospective trials (107,108) have contested these initial findings and supported the safety of letrozole compared to traditional ovulation induction treatment.

7. Oral contraceptives

Branigan & Estes., 2003 (109) in a RCT showed that the suppression of the hypothalamic pituitary- ovarian axis for 2 months with combined oral contraceptives (COC) (0.03 mg of ethinyl estradiol and 0.15 mg of desogestrel) followed by CC, at dosage of 100 mg/day on days fifth to ninth of the cycle, improved ovulation and pregnancy rates in CC resistant women in comparison with repeated cycles of CC alone. Oral contraceptive administration showed to reduce serum LH, estradiol and androgen levels. These hormonal changes, especially the reduced androgenic milieu, could act improving the ovarian microenvironment, and thus the ovarian response to CC. Kriplani et al., 2010 (110) in a RCT reported that in women with PCOS, a drospirenone containing COC has better outcome in terms of persistent regular cycles, antiandrogenic effect,fall in BMI and BP, better lipid profile, favorable glycemic and hormonal profile than desogestrel-containing COC.

8. N-acetyl-cysteine

N-acetyl-cysteine (NAC) is a mucolytic drug. Fulghesu et al., 2002 (111) demonstrated that long term NAC treatment (1.8 g/d for 5-6 weeks) was associated with significant increase in insulin sensitivity and reduction in insulin levels, testosterone and FAI in hyperinsulinemic PCOS. Rizk et al., 2005 (112) showed that the combination of NAC (1.2 g/d) with CC (100 mg/d) for only 5 days significantly increased both ovulation and pregnancy rates in obese women with CC-resistant PCOS compared with placebo (49.3% vs. 1.3% and 21.3% vs. 0, respectively). Actually, these results supporting the shorter duration (5 days only) of NAC administration in CC- resistant PCOS women have not been replicated by other trials. Recently, in a well designed adequately powered RCT, we reported that the efficacy of metformin–CC combination therapy is higher than that of NAC - CC for inducing ovulation and achieving pregnancy among CC-resistant PCOS patients (113). In our study, the dose and duration of NAC were chosen based on that published by Fulghesu et al., 2002(111). Over a 3-month follow-up period, women in metformin-CC group had significantly higher ovulation and pregnancy rates compared with women in NAC-CC group (69.1% vs. 20.0% and 22.7% vs. 5.3%, respectively). Moreover, the level of serum estrogen, the endometrial thickness on the day of hCG administration and the midluteal serum progesterone level were all significantly higher for women in metformin-CC group than other group. Additionally, a lower miscarriage rate was observed among women in metformin-CC group (113).

9. Dexamethasone therapy

Dexamethasone therapy during the follicular phase has been described without any side effects or serious events (114). Parsanezhad et al., 2002 (115) in a double-blind RCT, showed the safety and the efficacy of a high-dose short course of dexamethasone for inducing ovulation in 230 CC-resistant patients with PCOS and normal DHEAS levels. They reported significantly higher ovulation and pregnancy rates in those who received 200mg of CC (days 5-9) and 2mg of dexamethasone (days 5-14) compared with CC alone (88% vs. 20% and 40.5 vs. 4.2% respectively). In these patients, dexamethasone reduced circulating DHEAS, T, and LH levels and the LH/FSH ratio after 2 weeks of treatment (115). These results were further confirmed in another RCT (116).

10. Bromocriptine

Currently, evidence suggests that PCOS and hyperprolactinaemia are two distinct entities without a patho-physiological link (117-119). Bromocriptine administration provided no benefit in CC-resistant PCOS patients with normal prolactin levels, receiving 150mg CC (days 5–9) and bromocriptin continuously administrated at a dosage of 7.5 mg daily (120). On the contrary, the use of cabergoline, a long-acting ergoline D2 agonist derivative, has been proved to improve ovarian response in hyperprolactinemic patients with PCOS candidates for treatment with gonadaotrophins (121). These data suggested the presence of a dopaminergic component in the control of LH release in PCOS patients (121).

11. Conclusion

Ovulation induction in women with PCOS who present with CC-resistant anovulatory infertility remains a major challenge in gynecologic endocrinology. Traditional alternatives for CC-resistant patients include gonadotrophin therapy and laparoscopic ovarian diathermy. However, because of the cost and risk inherent in these therapies, alternative treatments are attractive. Obese PCOS women should try to attain BMI<30kg/m2 prior to commencing ovulation induction therapy. In view of our experience, combined metformin-CC therapy did result in modest ovulation and pregnancy rates. Accordingly, it is logical to offer combined metformin- CC therapy for CC-resistant PCOS patients before resorting to more expensive alternatives especially in developing communities where economic aspects of therapy are important. Third generation aromatase inhibitors are promising agents for treatment in these patients. Figure 1 shows an algorithm for ovulation induction treatment in anovulatory infertile women with CC-resistant PCOS.

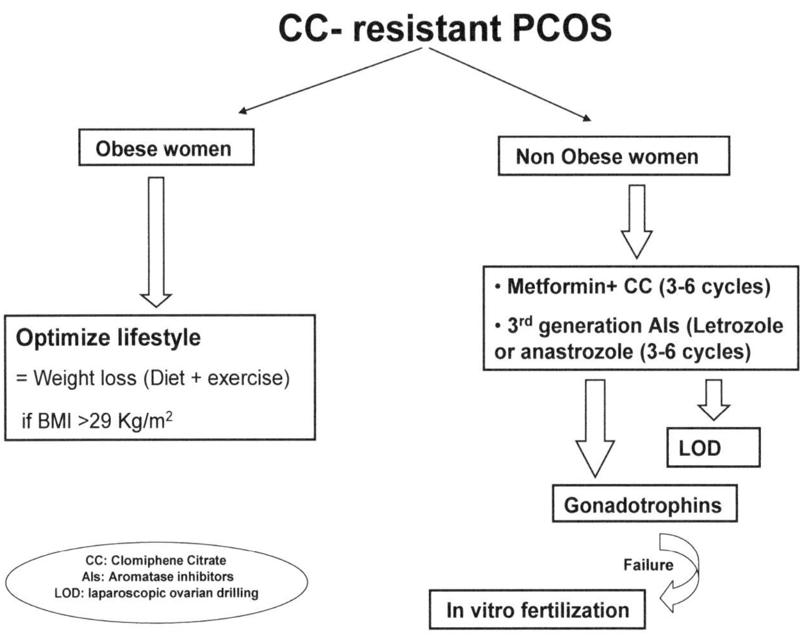

Fig. 1. Algorithm for ovulation induction treatment in anovulatory infertile women with CC-resistant PCOS.

12. References

[1] Overbeek, A. & Lambalk, CB. (2009). Phenotypic and pharmacogenetic aspects of ovulation induction in WHO II anovulatory women. Gynecological Endocrinology, Vol.25, No.4 , pp. 222–234

[2] Brown, J.; Farquhar, C.; Beck, J.; Boothroyd, C. & Hughes, E. (2009). Clomiphene and anti-oestrogens for ovulation induction in PCOS. Cochrane Database of Systematic Reviews, Issue 4. Art. No. CD002249.

[3] Diamanti-Kandarakis, E.; Kouli, CR.; Bergiele, AT.; Filandra, FA.; Tsianateli, TC.; Spina, GG.; Zapanti, ED. & Bartzis, MI. (1999). A survey of the polycystic ovary syndrome in the Greek island of Lesbos: hormonal and metabolic profile. The Journal of Clinical Endocrinology & Metabolism, Vol.84, No. 11, pp.4006-4011.

[4] Knochenhauer, ES.; Key, TJ.; Kahsar-Miller, M.; Waggoner, W.; Boots, LR. & Azziz, R. (1998). Prevalence of the polycystic ovary syndrome in unselected black and white women of the southeastern United States: a prospective study. The Journal of Clinical Endocrinology & Metabolism, Vol.83, No.9, pp. 3078-3082.

[5] Asuncion, M.; Calvo, RM.; San Millan, JL.; Sancho, J.; Avila, S. & Escobar-Morreale, HF. (2000). A prospective study of the prevalence of the polycystic ovary syndrome in unselected Caucasian women from Spain. The Journal of Clinical Endocrinology & Metabolism, Vol.85, No. 7, pp. 2434-2438.

[6] Azziz, R.; Woods, KS.; Reyna, R.; Key, TJ.; Knochenhauer, ES. & Yildiz, BO. (2004). The prevalence and features of the polycystic ovary syndrome in an unselected population. The Journal of Clinical Endocrinology & Metabolism, Vol.89, No. 6, pp. 2745-2749.

[7] March, WA.; Moore, VM.; Willson, KJ.; Phillips, DI.; Norman, RJ. & Davies, MJ. (2010). The prevalence of polycystic ovary syndrome in a community sample assessed under contrasting diagnostic criteria. Human Reproduction, Vol.25, No. 2, pp. 544-551.

[8] Thessaloniki ESHRE/ASRM-Sponsored PCOS Consensus Workshop Group. (2008). Consensus on infertility treatment related to polycystic ovary syndrome. Fertility and Sterility, Vol.89, No.3 ,pp.505-522

[9] Vause, TD.; Cheung, AP.; Sierra, S.; Claman, P.; Graham, J.; Guillemin, JA.; Lapensée, L.; Stewart, S.; Wong, BC. & Society of Obstetricians and Gynecologists of Canada. (2010). Ovulation induction in polycystic ovary syndrome. Journal of Obstetrics and Gynaecology Canada, Vol.32, No.5, pp. 495-502.

[10] Homburg, R. (2005). Clomiphene citrate-end of an era? A mini-review. Human Reproduction, Vol. 20, No.8, pp. 2043–2051.

[11] Imani, B.; Eijkemans, MJ.; te Velde, ER.; Habbema, JD. & Fauser, BC. (2002). A nomogram to predict the probability of live birth after clomiphene citrate induction of ovulation in normogonadotropic oligoamenorrheic infertility. Fertility and Sterility, Vol.77, No.1, pp. 91–97.

[12] Legro, RS.; Barnhart, HX.; Schlaff, WD.; Carr, BR.; Diamond, MP.; Carson, SA.; et al., & Cooperative Multicenter Reproductive Medicine Network. (2007). Clomiphene, metformin, or both for infertility in the polycystic ovary syndrome. The new England Journal of Medicine, Vol. 356, No. 6,pp.551–566

[13] National Collaborating Centre for Women's and Children's Health / National Institue for Clinical Excellence. (2004). Fertility: assessment and treatment for people with fertility problems. Clinical Guideline No. 11, RCOG Press, London, UK.
[14] Imani, B.; Eijkemans, MJC.; te Velde, ER.; Habbema, JD. & Fauser, BC. (1998). Predictors of patients remaining anovulatory during clomiphene citrate induction of ovulation in normogonadotropic oligoamenorrheic infertility. The Journal of Clinical Endocrinology & Metabolism, Vol.83, No.7, pp. 2361-2365.
[15] Imani, B.; Eijkemans, MJ.; de Jong, FH.; Payne, NN.; Bouchard, P.; Giudice, LC. & Fauser, B. (2000). Free androgen index and leptin are the most prominent endocrine predictors of ovarian response during clomiphene citrate induction of ovulation in normogonadotropic oligoamenorrheic infertility. The Journal of Clinical Endocrinology & Metabolism, Vol.85, No.2, pp. 676-682.
[16] Parsanezhad, ME.; Alborzi, S.; Zarei, A.; Dehbashi, S. & Omrani, G. (2001). Insulin resistance in clomiphene responders and nonresponders with polycystic ovarian disease and therapeutic effects of metformin. International Journal of Gynecology & Obstetrics, Vol.75, No.1, pp.43-50.
[17] Overbeek, A.; Kuijper, EA.; Hendriks, ML.; Blankenstein, M.A.; Ketel, I.J.; Twisk,J.W.; Hompes, P.G.; Homburg, R. & Lambalk, C.B. (2009). Clomiphene citrate resistance in relation to follicle-stimulating hormone receptor Ser680Ser-polymorphism in polycystic ovary syndrome. Human Reproduction, Vol.24, No.8 , pp. 2007-2013
[18] Al-Azemi, M.; Omu, F.E. & Omu, A.E. (2004). The effect of obesity on the outcome of infertility management in women with polycystic ovary syndrome. Archives of Gynecology and Obstetrics, Vol. 270, No.4, pp.205-210.
[19] Norman, RJ.; Noakes, M.; Wu, R.; Davies, MJ.; Moran, L. & Wang, JX. (2004). Improving reproductive performance in overweight/obese women with effective weight management. Human Reproduction Update, Vol.10, No.3 ,pp. 267-280.
[20] Norman, RJ.; Davies, MJ.; Lord, J. & Moran, LJ. (2002). The role of lifestyle modification in polycystic ovary syndrome. Trends in Endocrinology and Metabolism, Vol.13, No. 6, pp.251-257.
[21] Hoeger, K.M. (2007). Obesity and lifestyle management in polycystic ovary syndrome. Clinical Obstetrics and Gynecology, Vol.50, No. 1, pp.277-294.
[22] Pasquali, R.; Gambineri, A. & Pagotto, U. (2006). The impact of obesity on reproduction in women with polycystic ovary syndrome. British Journal of Obstetrics & Gynaecology, Vol.113, No.10, pp.1148-1159.
[23] Tolino, A.; Gambardella, V.; Caccavale, C.; D'Ettore, A.; Giannotti, F.; D'Anto, V. & De Falco, C.L. (2005). Evaluation of ovarian functionality after a dietary treatment in obese women with polycystic ovary syndrome. European Journal of Obstetrics & Gynecology and Reproductive Biology, Vol. 119, No.1, pp. 87-93.
[24] Moran, LJ.; Pasquali, R.; Teede, HJ.; Hoeger, KM. & Norman, RJ. (2009). Treatment of obesity in polycystic ovary syndrome: a position statement of the Androgen Excess and Polycystic Ovary Syndrome Society. Fertility and Sterility, Vol. 92, No.6, pp.1966-1982.
[25] Moran, LJ.; Hutchison, SK.; Norman, RJ. & Teede, HJ. (2011). Lifestyle changes in women with polycystic ovary syndrome. Cochrane Database of Systematic Reviews, Issue 2. Art. No.CD007506.

[26] Stamets, K.; Taylor, DS.; Kunselman, A.; Demers, LM.; Pelkman, CL. & Legro, RS. (2004). A randomized trial of the effects of two types of short-term hypocaloric diets on weight loss in women with polycystic ovary syndrome. Fertility and Sterility, Vol.81, No. 3, pp. 630–637.

[27] Moran, LJ.; Noakes, M.; Clifton, PM.; Tomlinson, L. & Norman, RJ. (2003). Dietary composition in restoring reproductive and metabolic physiology in overweight women with polycystic ovary syndrome. The Journal of Clinical Endocrinology & Metabolism, Vol.88, No.2, pp.812–819.

[28] Poehlman, ET.; Dvorak, RV.; DeNino, WF.; Brochu, M. & Ades, PA. (2000). Effects of resistance training and endurance training on insulin sensitivity in nonobese, young women: a controlled randomized trial. The Journal of Clinical Endocrinology & Metabolism, Vol.85, No.7, pp. 2463-2468.

[29] Palomba, S.; Falbo, A.; Giallauria, F.; Russo, T.; Rocca, M.; Tolino, A.; Zullo, F. & Orio, F. (2010). Six weeks of structured exercise training and hypocaloric diet increases the probability of ovulation after clomiphene citrate in overweight and obese patients with polycystic ovary syndrome: a randomized controlled trial. Human Reproduction, Vol.25, No. 11, pp. 2783-2791.

[30] Otta, CF.; Wior, M.; Iraci, GS.; Kaplan, R.; Torres, D.; Gaido, MI. & Wyse, EP. (2010). Clinical, metabolic, and endocrine parameters in response to metformin and lifestyle intervention in women with polycystic ovary syndrome: a randomized, double-blind, and placebo control trial. Gynecological Endocrinology, Vol.26, No.3, pp. 173-178.

[31] Karimzadeh, MA. & Javedani, M. (2010). An assessment of lifestyle modification versus medical treatment with clomiphene citrate, metformin, and clomiphene citrate-metformin in patients with polycystic ovary syndrome. Fertility and Sterility, Vol.94, No.1, pp.216-220.

[32] Alvarez-Blasco, F.; Botella-Carretero, J.I.; San Millán, J.L.& Escobar-Morreale, H.F. (2006). Prevalence and characteristics of the polycystic ovary syndrome in overweight and obese women. Archives of Internal Medicine. Vol. 166, No.19, pp.2081-2086.

[33] Escobar-Morreale, H.F.; Botella-Carretero, J.I.; Alvarez-Blasco, F.; Sancho, J. & San Millán, J.L. (2005). The polycystic ovary syndrome associated with morbid obesity may resolve after weight loss induced by bariatric surgery. The Journal of Clinical Endocrinology & Metabolism, Vol. 90, No. 12, pp.6364-6369.

[34] Jayagopal, V.; Kilpatrick, E.S.; Holding, S.; Jennings, P.E. & Atkin, S.L. (2005). Orlistat is as beneficial as metformin in the treatment of polycystic ovarian syndrome. The Journal of Clinical Endocrinology & Metabolism, Vol. 90, No.2, pp.729–733.

[35] Sabuncu, T.; Harma, M.; Nazligul, Y. & Kilic, F. (2003). Sibutramine has a positive effect on clinical and metabolic parameters in obese patients with polycystic ovary syndrome. Fertility and Sterility, Vol. 80, No. 5, pp. 1199–1204.

[36] Cristello, F.; Cela, V.; Artini, PG. & Genazzani, AR. (2005). Therapeutic strategies for ovulation induction in infertile women with polycystic ovary syndrome. Gynecological Endocrinology, Vol.21, No. 6, pp. 340–352.

[37] Ratts, VS.; Pauls, RN.; Pinto, AB.; Kraja, A.; Williams, DB. & Odem, RR. (2007). Risk of multiple gestation after ovulation induction in polycystic ovary syndrome. The Journal of Reproductive Medicine, Vol.52, No.10, pp. 896–900.

[38] Yarali, H. & Zeyneloglu, HB. (2004). Gonadotrophin treatment in patients with polycystic ovary syndrome. Reproductive BioMedicine Online, Vol.8, No. 5 ,pp.528-537.

[39] Tummon, I.; Gavrilova-Jordan, L.; Allemand, MC. & Session, D. (2005) Polycystic ovaries and ovarian hyperstimulation syndrome: a systematic review. Acta Obstetricia et Gynecologica Scandinavica, Vol. 84, No.7, pp. 611–616.

[40] Van der Meer, M,; Hompes, P.; de Boer, J.; Schats, R. & Schoemaker, J. (1998). Cohort size rather than follicle-stimulating hormone threshold levels determines ovarian sensitivity in polycystic ovary syndrome. The Journal of Clinical Endocrinology & Metabolism, Vol.83, No.2, pp. 423–426.

[41] Nugent, D.; Vandekerckhove, P.; Hughes, E.; Arnot, M. & Lilford, R. (2000) Gonadotrophin therapy for ovulation induction in subfertility associated with polycystic ovary syndrome. Cochrane Database of Systematic Reviews, Issue 4. Art. No. CD000410.

[42] Homburg, R. & Insler, V. (2002). Ovulation induction in perspective. Human Reproduction Update, Vol.8, No.5, pp.449 - 462.

[43] Homburg, R. & Howles, CM. (1999). Low-dose FSH therapy for anovulatory infertility associated with polycystic ovary syndrome: rationale, reflections and refinements. Human Reproduction Update, Vol.5, No.5 ,pp.493–499.

[44] White, DM.; Polson, DW.; Kiddy, D.; Sagle, P.; Watson, H.; Gilling-Smith, C.; Hamilton-Fairley, D. & Franks, S. (1996). Induction of ovulation with low-dose gonadotropins in polycystic ovary syndrome: an analysis of 109 pregnancies in 225 women. The Journal of Clinical Endocrinology & Metabolism, Vol.81, No.11, pp. 3821-3824.

[45] Bayram, N.; van Wely, M. & van der Veen, F. (2001). Recombinant FSH versus urinary gonadotrophins or recombinant FSH for ovulation induction in subfertility associated with polycystic ovarian syndrome. Cochrane Database of Systematic Reviews, Issue 2. Art. No. CD002121.

[46] van Wely, M.; Bayram, N. & van der Veen, F (2003). Recombinant FSH in alternative doses or versus urinary gonadotrophins for ovulation induction in subfertility associated with polycystic ovary syndrome: a systematic review based on a Cochrane review. Human Reproduction, Vol.18, No.6, pp.1143-1149.

[47] Balen, A.; Platteau, P.; Andersen, AN.; Devroey, P.; Helmgaard, L.& Arce, J-C. (2007). Highly purified FSH is as efficacious as recombinant FSH for ovulation induction in women with WHO Group II anovulatory infertility: a randomized controlled non-inferiority trial. Human Reproduction, Vol.22, No.7, pp.1816–1823.

[48] Farquhar, C.M.; Williamson, K.; Gudex, G.; Johnson, N.P.; Garland, J. & Sadler, L. (2002). A randomized controlled trial of laparoscopic ovarian diathermy versus gonadotropin therapy for women with clomiphene citrate resistant polycystic ovary syndrome. Fertility and Sterility, Vol.78, No.2, pp. 404-411.

[49] Farquhar, C.; Lilford, RJ.; Marjoribanks, J. & Vandekerckhove, P. (2007). Laparoscopic 'drilling' by diathermy or laser for ovulation induction in anovulatory polycystic ovary syndrome. Cochrane Database of Systematic Reviews, Issue 3. Art. No. CD001122.

[50] Bayram, N.; van Wely, M.; Kaaijk, EM.; Bossuyt, PM. & van der Veen, F. (2004). Using an electrocautery strategy or recombinant follicle stimulating hormone to induce

ovulation in polycystic ovary syndrome: randomised controlled trial. British Medical Journal, Vol.328 (7433):192.
[51] Flyckt, RL. & Goldberg, JM. (2011). Laparoscopic ovarian drilling for clomiphene-resistant polycystic ovary syndrome. Seminars in Reproductive Medicine. Vol.29, No.2, pp.138-146.
[52] Nahuis, MJ.; Kose, N.; Bayram, N.; van Dessel, HJ.; Braat, DD.; Hamilton, CJ.; Hompes, PG.; Bossuyt, PM.; Mol, BW.; van der Veen, F. & van Wely, M. (2011). Long-term outcomes in women with polycystic ovary syndrome initially randomized to receive laparoscopic electrocautery of the ovaries or ovulation induction with gonadotrophins.. Human Reproduction, Vol. 26, No.7, pp.1899-1904.
[53] Felemban, A.; Lin Tan, S. & Tulandi, T. (2000). Laparoscopic treatment of polycystic ovaries with insulated needle cautery: a reappraisal. Fertility and Sterility, Vol.73, No.2, pp. 266–269.
[54] Mercorio, F.; Mercorio, A.; Di Spiezio Sardo, A.; Barba, GV.; Pellicano, M. & Nappi, C. (2008). Evaluation of ovarian adhesion formation after laparoscopic ovarian drilling by second-look minilaparoscopy. Fertility and Sterility, Vol.89, No. 5, pp. 1229-1233.
[55] Api, M. (2009). Is ovarian reserve diminished after laparoscopic ovarian drilling? Gynecological Endocrinology, Vol.25, No.3, pp. 159-165.
[56] Farquhar, CM.; Williamson, K.; Brown, PM. & Garland, J. (2004). An economic evaluation of laparoscopic ovarian diathermy versus gonadotrophin therapy for women with clomiphene citrate resistant polycystic ovary syndrome. Human Reproduction, Vol.19, No.5, pp.1110-1115.
[57] Amer, S.; Li, TC.; & Cooke, ID. (2003). A prospective dose finding study of the amount of energy required for laparoscopic ovarian diathermy in women with polycystic ovarian syndrome. Human Reproduction, Vol.18, No.8, pp.1693–1698.
[58] Roy, KK.; Baruah, J.; Moda, N. & Kumar, S. (2009). Evaluation of unilateral versus bilateral ovarian drilling in clomiphene citrate resistant cases of polycystic ovarian syndrome. Archives of Gynecology and Obstetrics, Vol. 280, No.4, pp.573-578.
[59] Al-Mizyen, E. & Grudzinskas, JG. (2007). Unilateral laparoscopic ovarian diathermy in infertile women with clomiphene citrate-resistant polycystic ovary syndrome. Fertility and Sterility, Vol. 88, No.6, pp.1678-1680.
[60] Youssef, H. & Atallah, MM. (2007). Unilateral ovarian drilling in polycystic ovarian syndrome: a prospective randomized study. Reproductive BioMedicine Online, Vol.15, No.4, pp.457-462.
[61] Kato, M.; Kikuchi, I.; Shimaniki, H.; Kobori, H.; Aida, T.; Kitade, M.; Kumakiri, J. & Takeuchi, H. (2007). Efficacy of laparoscopic ovarian drilling for polycystic ovary syndrome resistant to clomiphene citrate. The Journal of Obstetrics and Gynaecology Research,Vol. 33, No.2,pp.174-180.
[62] Seow, KM.; Juan, CC.; Hwang, JL. & Ho, LT. (2008). Laparoscopic surgery in polycystic ovary syndrome: reproductive and metabolic effects. Seminars in Reproductive Medicine, Vol. 26, No.1, pp.101-110.
[63] Amer, SA.; Li, TC. & Ledger, WL. (2004). Ovulation induction using laparoscopic ovarian drilling in women with polycystic ovarian syndrome: predictors of success. Human Reproduction, Vol.19, No. 8, pp.1719-1724.

[64] van Wely, .; Bayram, N.; van der Veen, F. & Bossuyt, PM. (2005). Predictors for treatment failure after laparoscopic electrocautery of the ovaries in women with clomiphene citrate resistant polycystic ovary syndrome. Human Reproduction, Vol.20, No. 4, pp.900-905.

[65] Mohiuddin, S.; Bessellink, D. & Farquhar, C. (2007). Long-term follow up of women with laparoscopic ovarian diathermy for women with clomiphene resistant polycystic ovarian syndrome. The Australian and New Zealand Journal of Obstetrics and Gynaecology , Vol. 47, No. 6, pp.508-511.

[66] Abu Hashim, H.; El-Shafei, M.; Badawy, A.; Wafa, A. & Zaglol, H. (2011). Does laparoscopic ovarian diathermy change clomiphene-resistant PCOS into clomiphene-sensitive? Archives of Gynecology and Obstetrics, Vol. 284, No. 2, pp.503-507.

[67] Legro, RS.; Castracane, VD. & Kauffman, RP. (2004). Detecting insulin resistance in polycystic ovary syndrome: purposes and pitfalls. Obstetrical And Gynecological Survey, Vol. 59, No. 2 , pp.141–154.

[68] Diamanti-Kandarakis, E.; Christakou, CD.; Kandaraki, E. & Economou, FN. (2010). Metformin: an old medication of new fashion: evolving new molecular mechanisms and clinical implications in polycystic ovary syndrome. European Journal of Endocrinology, Vol.162, No.2, pp.193-212.

[69] Johnson, N. (2011). Metformin is a reasonable first-line treatment option for non-obese women with infertility related to anovulatory polycystic ovary syndrome--a meta-analysis of randomised trials. The Australian and New Zealand Journal of Obstetrics and Gynaecology , Vol.51, No. 2, pp.125-129.

[70] Tang, T.; Lord, JM.; Norman, RJ.; Yasmin, E. & Balen, AH. (2010). Insulin-sensitising drugs (metformin, rosiglitazone, pioglitazone, D-chiro-inositol) for women with polycystic ovary syndrome, oligo amenorrhoea and subfertility. Cochrane Database of Systematic Reviews, Issue 1. Art. No. CD003053.

[71] Nesler, JE.; Jakubowicz, DJ.; Evans, WS. & Pasquali, R. (1998). Effects of metformin on spontaneous and clomiphene-induced ovulation in the polycystic ovary syndrome. The new England Journal of Medicine, Vol. 338, No. 26, pp.1876–1880.

[72] Vandermolen, DT.; Ratts, V.; Evans, WS.; Stovall, DW.; Kauma, SW. & Nester, JE. (2001). Metformin increases the ovulatory rate and pregnancy rate from clomiphene citrate in patient with polycystic ovary syndrome who is resistant to clomiphene citrate alone. Fertility and Sterility, Vol.75, No. 2 , pp.310 –315.

[73] Kocak, M.; Caliskan, E.; Simsir, C. & Haberal, A. (2002). Metformin therapy improves ovulatory rates, cervical scores, and pregnancy rates in clomiphene citrate–resistant women with polycystic ovary syndrome. Fertility and Sterility, Vol. 77, No. 1, pp.101- 106.

[74] Creanga, AA.; Bradley, HM.; McCormick, C. & Witkop, CT. (2008). Use of metformin in polycystic ovary syndrome: a meta-analysis. Obstetrics & Gynecology, Vol.111, No.4, pp.959-968.

[75] Attia, GR.; Rainey, WE. & Bruce, RC. (2001). Metformin directly inhibits androgen production in human thecal cells. Fertility and Sterility, Vol. 76, No. 3 pp.517–524.

[76] la Marca, A.; Morgante, G.; Paglia, T.; Ciotta, L.; Cianci, A. & De Leo, V. (1999). Effects of metformin on adrenal steroidogenesis in women with polycystic ovary syndrome. Fertility and Sterility, Vol. 72, No. 6, pp.985-989.

[77] Billa, E.; Kapolla, N.; Nicopoulou, SC.; Koukkou, E.; Venaki, E.; Milingos, S.; Antsaklis, A. & Adamopoulos, D.A. (2009). Metformin administration was associated with a modification of LH, prolactin and insulin secretion dynamics in women with polycystic ovarian syndrome. Gynecological Endocrinology, Vol. 25, No. 7, pp.427-434.

[78] Palomba, S.; Falbo, A.; Battista, L.; Russo, T.; Venturella, R.; Tolino, A.; Orio, F. & Zullo, F. (2010). Laparoscopic ovarian diathermy vs clomiphene citrate plus metformin as second-line strategy for infertile anovulatory patients with polycystic ovary syndrome: a randomized controlled trial. American Journal of Obstetrics and Gynecology, Vol. 202, No. 6,pp.577.e1-8.

[79] Abu Hashim, H.; El Lakany, N. & Sherief, L. (2011). Combined metformin and clomiphene citrate versus laparoscopic ovarian diathermy for ovulation induction in clomiphene-resistant women with polycystic ovary syndrome: A randomized controlled trial. The Journal of Obstetrics and Gynaecology Research, Vol.37, No. 3, pp.169-177.

[80] George, SS.; George, K.; Irwin, C.; Job, V.; Selvakumar, R.; Jeyaseelan, V. & Seshadri, M.S. (2003). Sequential treatment of metformin and clomiphene citrate in clomiphene-resistant women with polycystic ovary syndrome: a randomized, controlled trial. Human Reproduction, Vol.18, No. 2, pp.299-304.

[81] Abu Hashim, H.; Wafa, A. & El Rakhawy, M. (2011). Combined metformin and clomiphene citrate versus highly purified FSH for ovulation induction in clomiphene-resistant PCOS women: a randomised controlled trial. Gynecological Endocrinology, Vol.27, No. 3, pp.190-196.

[82] Gilbert, C.; Valois, M. & Koren, G. (2006). Pregnancy outcome after first-trimester exposure to metformin: a meta-analysis. Fertility and Sterility, Vol. 86, No. 3, pp. 658-663.

[83] Ijäs,H.; Vääräsmäki, M.; Morin-Papunen, L.; Keravuo, R.; Ebeling, T.; Saarela, T. & Raudaskoski T. (2011). Metformin should be considered in the treatment of gestational diabetes: a prospective randomised study. British Journal of Obstetrics & Gynaecology, Vol.118, No.7, pp. 880-885.

[84] Nawaz, F.H.; Khalid, R.; Naru, T. & Rizvi, J. (2008). Does continuous use of metformin throughout pregnancy improve pregnancy outcomes in women with polycystic ovarian syndrome? The Journal of Obstetrics and Gynaecology Research, Vol. 34, No. 4, pp.832-837.

[85] Rowan, J.A.; Hague, W.M.; Gao, W.; Battin, M.R.; Moore, M.P. & MiG Trial Investigators. (2008). Metformin versus insulin for the treatment of gestational diabetes. The new England Journal of Medicine, Vol. 358, No. 19, pp.2003-2015.

[86] Palomba, S.; Falbo, A.; Orio, F. Jr. & Zullo, F. (2009). Effect of preconceptional metformin on abortion risk in polycystic ovary syndrome: a systematic review and meta-analysis of randomized controlled trials. Fertility and Sterility, Vol. 92, No. 5, pp.1646-1658

[87] Rouzi, A.A. & Ardawi, M.S. (2006). A randomized controlled trial of the efficacy of rosiglitazone and clomiphene citrate versus metformin and clomiphene citrate in women with clomiphene citrate-resistant polycystic ovary syndrome. Fertility and Sterility, Vol.85, No. 2, pp.428–435.

[88] Roy, K.K.; Baruah, J.; Sharma, A.; Sharma, JB.; Kumar, S.; Kachava, G. & Karmakar, D.A. (2010). prospective randomized trial comparing the clinical and endocrinological outcome with rosiglitazone versus laparoscopic ovarian drilling in patients with polycystic ovarian disease resistant to ovulation induction with clomiphene citrate. Archives of Gynecology and Obstetrics, Vol. 281, No. 5, pp.939-944.

[89] Shokeir, T. & El-Kannishy, G. (2008). Rosiglitazone as treatment for clomiphene citrate-resistant polycystic ovary syndrome: factors associated with clinical response. Journal of Womens Health (Larchmt), Vol. 17, No. 9, pp.1445-1452.

[90] Mauri, D.; Pavlidis, N.; Polyzos, NP. & Ioannidis, JP. (2006). Survival with aromatase inhibitors and inactivators versus standard hormonal therapy in advanced breast cancer: meta-analysis. Journal of the National Cancer Institute. Vol. 98, No. 18, pp.1285-1291.

[91] Mitwally, M.F.M. & Casper, R.F. (2001). Use of an aromatase inhibitor for induction of ovulation in patients with an inadequate response to clomiphene citrate. Fertility and Sterility, Vol.75, No. 2, pp. 305-309.

[92] Casper, R.F. & Mitwally, M.F.M. (2006). Aromatase inhibitors for ovulation induction. The Journal of Clinical Endocrinology & Metabolism, Vol.91, No. 3, pp. 760-771.

[93] Begum, M.R.; Ferdous, J.; Begum, A. & Quadir, E. (2009). Comparison of efficacy of aromatase inhibitor and clomiphene citrate in induction of ovulation in polycystic ovarian syndrome. Fertility and Sterility, Vol. 92, No. 3, pp. 853-857.

[94] Kamath, M.S.; Aleyamma, T.K.; Chandy, A. George, k. (2010). Aromatase inhibitors in women with clomiphene citrate resistance: a randomized, double-blind, placebo-controlled trial. Fertility and Sterility, Vol. 94, No. 7, pp. 2857-2859.

[95] Pritts, EA. (2010). Letrozole for ovulation induction and controlled ovarian hyperstimulation. Current Opinion in Obstetrics and Gynecology, Vol. 22, No. 4 , pp.289-294.

[96] Lee, V.C.& Ledger, W. (2011). Aromatase inhibitors for ovulation induction and ovarian stimulation. Clinical Endocrinology (Oxf), Vol.74, No. 5, pp.537-546.

[97] Al-Omari, W.R.; Sulaiman, W. & Al-Hadithi, N. (2004). Comparison of two aromatase inhibitors in women with clomiphene-resistant polycystic ovary syndrome. International Journal of Gynecology & Obstetrics, Vol.85, No. 3 ,pp. 289-91.

[98] Badawy, A.; Mosbah, A. & Shady, M. (2008). Anastrozole or letrozole for ovulation induction in clomiphene-resistant women with polycystic ovarian syndrome: a prospective randomized trial. Fertility and Sterility, Vol. 89, No. 5, pp. 1209-1212.

[99] Badawy, A.; Mosbah, A.; Tharwat, A. & Eid, M. (2009). Extended letrozole therapy for ovulation induction in clomiphene-resistant women with polycystic ovary syndrome: a novel protocol. Fertility and Sterility, Vol. 92, No.1, pp.236-239.

[100] Sohrabvand, F.; Ansari, S. & Bagheri, M. (2006). Efficacy of combined metformin - letrozole in comparison with metformin - clomiphene in clomiphene resistant infertile women with polycystic ovary disease. Human Reproduction, Vol.21, No. 6, pp.1432 - 1435.

[101] Abu Hasim, H.; Shokeir, T. & Badawy, A. (2010). Letrozole versus combined metformin and clomiphene citrate for ovulation induction in clomiphene-resistant women with polycystic ovary syndrome: a randomized controlled trial. Fertility and Sterility, Vol.94, No. 4,pp. 1405-1409.

[102] Abu Hasim, H.; Mashaly, A. M. & Badawy, A. (2010). Letrozole versus laparoscopic ovarian diathermy for ovulation induction in clomiphene- resistant women with polycystic ovary syndrome: a randomized controlled trial. Archives of Gynecology and Obstetrics, Vol. 282, No. 5,pp. 567–571.

[103] Abdellah, M.S. (2011). Reproductive outcome after letrozole versus laparoscopic ovarian drilling for clomiphene-resistant polycystic ovary syndrome. International Journal of Gynecology & Obstetrics, Vol. 113, No. 3 pp. 218-221.

[104] Ganesh, A.; Goswami, S.K.; Chattopadhyay, R.; Chaudhury, K. & Chakravarty, B. (2009). Comparison of letrozole with continuous gonadotropins and clomiphene-gonadotropin combination for ovulation induction in 1387 PCOS women after clomiphene citrate failure: a randomized prospective clinical trial. Journal of Assisted Reproduction and Genetics , Vol. 26, No. 1, pp.19-24.

[105] Elnashar, A.; Fouad, H.; Eldosoky, M. & Saeid, N. (2006). Letrozole induction of ovulation in women with clomiphene citrate resistant polycystic ovary syndrome may not depend on the period of infertility, the body mass index, or the luteinizing hormone/follicle-stimulating hormone ratio. Fertility and Sterility, Vol. 85, No. 2, pp.511-513.

[106] Biljan, M.M.; Hemmings, R. & Brassard, N. (2005). The outcome of 150 babies following the treatment with letrozole or letrozole and gonadotropins. Fertility and Sterility, Vol. 84, Supplement 1, S95.

[107] Tulandi, T.; Martin, J.; Al-Fadhli, R.; Kabli, N.; Forman, R.; Hitkari, J.; Librach, C.; Greenblatt, E. & Casper, R.F. (2006). Congenital malformations among 911 newborns conceived after infertility treatment with letrozole or clomiphene citrate. Fertility and Sterility, Vol. 85, No. 6, pp.1761–1765.

[108] Badawy, A.; Shokeir, A.; Allam, A.F. & Abdelhady, H. (2009). Pregnancy outcome after ovulation induction with aromatase inhibitors or clomiphene citrate in unexplained infertility. Acta Obstetricia et Gynecologica Scandinavica, Vol. 88, No. 2, pp.187–191.

[109] Branigan, E.F. & Estes, M.A. (2003). A randomized clinical trial of treatment of clomiphene citrate-resistant anovulation with the use of oral contraceptive pill suppression and repeat clomiphene citrate treatment. American Journal of Obstetrics and Gynecology, Vol. 188, No. 6 ,pp.1424-1428..

[110] Kriplani, A.; Periyasamy, A.J.; Agarwal, N.; Kulshrestha, V. Kumar, A. & Ammini, A.C. (2010). Effect of oral contraceptive containing ethinyl estradiol combined with drospirenone vs. desogestrel on clinical and biochemical parameters in patients with polycystic ovary syndrome. Contraception, Vol. 82, No. 2, pp.139-146.

[111] Flughesu, A.M.; Ciampelli, M.; Muzj, G.; Belosi, C.; Selvaggi, L. & Ayala, G.F. (2002). N-acetyl cysteine treatment improves insulin sensitivity in women with polycystic ovary syndrome. Fertility and Sterility, Vol.77, No. 6, pp.1128 -1135.

[112] Rizk, A.; Bedaiwy, M. & Al-Inany, H. (2005). N-acetyl-cysteine is a novel adjuvant to clomiphene citrate in clomiphene citrate–resistant patients with polycystic ovary syndrome. Fertility and Sterility, Vol. 83, No. 2, pp.367–370.

[113] Abu Hashim, H.; Anwar, K. & El-Fatah, R.A. (2010). N-acetyl cysteine plus clomiphene citrate versus metformin and clomiphene citrate in treatment of clomiphene resistant polycystic ovary syndrome: a randomized controlled trial. Journal of Womens Health (Larchmt), Vol.19, No. 11, pp.2043-2048.

[114] Trott, E.A.; Plouffe, L. Jr.; Hansen, K.; Hines, R.; Brann, D.W. &Mahesh, V.B. (1996). Ovulation induction in clomiphene-resistant anovulatory women with normal dehydroepiandrosterone sulfate levels: beneficial effects of the addition of dexamethasone during the follicular phase. Fertility and Sterility, Vol. 66, No. 3, pp.484-486.

[115] Parsanezhad, M.E.; Alborzi, S.; Motazedian, S. & Omrani, G. (2002). Use of dexamethasone and clomiphene citrate in the treatment of clomiphene citrate-resistant patients with polycystic ovary syndrome and normal dehydroepiandrosterone sulfate levels: a prospective, double-blind, placebo-controlled trial. Fertility and Sterility, Vol.78, No. 5, pp.1001-1004.

[116] Elnashar, A.; Abdelmageed, E.; Fayed, M. & Sharaf, M. (2006). Clomiphene citrate and dexamethazone in treatment of clomiphene citrate-resistant polycystic ovary syndrome: a prospective placebo-controlled study. Human Reproduction. Vol.21, No. 7, pp.1805-1808.

[117] Filho, R.B.; Domingues, L.; Naves, L.; Ferraz, E.; Alves, A. & Casulari, L.A. (2007). Polycystic ovary syndrome and hyperprolactinemia are distinct entities. Gynecological Endocrinology, Vol. 23, No.5, pp.267-272.

[118] Su, H.W.; Chen, C.M.; Chou, S.Y.; Liang, S.J.; Hsu, C.S. & Hsu, M.I. (2011) . Polycystic ovary syndrome or hyperprolactinaemia: a study of mild hyperprolactinaemia. Gynecological Endocrinology, Vol. 27, No.1, pp.55-62.

[119] Robin, G.; Catteau-Jonard, S.; Young, J. & Dewailly, D. (2011). Physiopathological link between polycystic ovary syndrome and hyperprolactinemia: myth or reality?. Gynécologie Obstétrique & Fertilité. Vol. 39, No.3, pp.141-145.

[120] Parsanezhad, M.E.; Alborzi, S. & Namavar Jahromi B. (2004). A prospective, double-blind, randomized, placebo-controlled clinical trial of bromocriptin in clomiphene-resistant patients with polycystic ovary syndrome and normal prolactin level. Archives of Gynecology and Obstetrics, Vol. 269, No.2 ,pp.125-129.

[121] Papaleo, E.; Doldi, N.; De Santis, L.; Marelli, G.; Marsiglio, E.; Rofena, S. & Ferrari, A. (2001). Cabergoline influences ovarian stimulation in hyperprolactinaemic patients with polycystic ovary syndrome. Human Reproduction. Vol. 16, No.11, pp.2263-2266.

2

Psycho-Social and Sexual Well-Being in Women with Polycystic Ovary Syndrome

J.E. de Niet[1,2], H. Pastoor[1], R. Timman[2] and J.S.E. Laven[1]
[1]*Division of Reproductive Medicine, Department of Obstetrics and Gynaecology, Erasmus MC University Medical Centre, Rotterdam,*
[2]*Department of Medical Psychology and Psychotherapy, Erasmus MC University Medical Centre, Rotterdam, Netherlands*

1. Introduction

The polycystic ovary syndrome (PCOS) is the most common endocrine disorder in women of reproductive age [1]. PCOS is not only accompanied with negative physical consequences, but this syndrome also affects psycho-social and sexual well-being. Characteristics of PCOS include enlarged ovaries with a polycystic appearance along with menstrual irregularities such as amenorrhoea or oligoamenorrhoea, excessive growth of body hair (hirsutism) or biochemical hyperandrogenism, and to a lesser extent acne. In addition, PCOS is associated with anovulatory infertility, obesity, insulin resistance, and lipid disorders [2, 3].

In clinical scenarios, the treatment of women with PCOS is mainly focused on correcting menstrual disturbances and physical consequences. Besides the physical consequences, the negative implications of PCOS in daily life such as impaired social contacts and sexual satisfaction and depression seem to be rarely discussed with PCOS women during treatment. The scientific interest in the psycho-social and sexual consequences of PCOS has grown in the past years and has increased our knowledge on these topics. For example, recent studies indicated that PCOS is associated with depression [4-6], body dissatisfaction [5, 6], decreased quality of life [7], a decreased feeling of sexual attractiveness and self-esteem as well as sexual dissatisfaction [4, 7].

First, an extensive overview is provided in this chapter on what is known about psycho-social and sexual well-being in women with PCOS (Part I). Second, we studied the association between on the one hand common physical features of PCOS (polycystic ovaries, hirsutism, acne, menstrual irregularities, and Body Mass Index) and endocrine variables (e.g. testosterone, progesterone, and estradiol) and sexual well-being on the other hand (Part II). In addition, we evaluated whether there is an association between aspects of psycho-social well-being (self-esteem, body satisfaction, and self-perceived fear of negative appearance evaluation) and sexual well-being (Part II).

2. Part I: Psycho-social well-being in women with PCOS

In some women, the appearance of PCOS might be characterized by an excess growth of body hair on various body areas such as the chin, lip, abdomen, and arms as well as by acne. It is imaginable that these outer appearances, together with non-visible characteristics (e.g. menstrual irregularities) influence psycho-social well-being. Moreover, PCOS causes infertility and involuntary childlessness. It has in fact been shown that women with PCOS report more psychological distress than controls [7, 8]. With respect to the diagnosis of PCOS itself, one study measuring patient's perception of the diagnosis of PCOS found that the emotions associated with the diagnosis included frustration (67%), anxiety (16%), and sadness (10%) [9].

It has been shown that hirsutism, menstrual irregularities, and infertility are the PCOS symptoms experienced as most bothersome by affected women [10]. Lipton and colleagues [11] demonstrated that women with facial hair spend a considerable time on the management of their facial hair (104 min/week). Besides, two thirds reported continually checking their facial hair in mirrors and 76% by touch. In addition, more than half of the women tried at least four methods for hair removal in the past. Furthermore, it is conceivable that infertility increases a woman's emotional distress. Indeed, many PCOS women seem to worry about remaining without children in the future and report a current wish to conceive; however, infertility does not appear to be a determinant for psychological problems [12]. Together, it is imaginable that the symptoms of PCOS might cause a woman to experience issues with their femininity and might therefore not only affect psychological well-being, but more in particular sexual well-being. Studies have indicated that women with PCOS experience more psychological problems such as depression and anxiety than non-PCOS controls with infertility problems [13], indicating that mood swings might be caused by the distressing symptoms of the syndrome. The emotional distress related to symptoms and consequences of PCOS might affect various domains of their lives, including romantic relationships, friendships, social contacts, and their working life. It could be that women find it difficult to share their experiences with other people and feel uncomfortable when conversations about motherhood are started. Also, about 50% of all women with PCOS are overweight, compared to 30% of women in the general population [2]. A higher Body Mass Index (BMI) in women with PCOS is not only related to negative physical [2, 3, 14, 15], but also to negative psychological consequences [4].

Altogether, a greater incidence of psychological problems have been found in women with PCOS [8]. In the sections below we will describe what is known about psycho-social well-being in women with PCOS as well as the association with features of PCOS. The results will not be discussed in detail as this is beyond the scope of this chapter.

2.1 Quality of Life

It is widely recognized that QoL is significantly reduced in women with PCOS [6, 16-18]. Generic QoL (focuses on domains of well-being in general) [19, 20] as well as specific QoL (focuses on domains of well-being related to a specific disease/syndrome) measurements [21] are used in research. Several studies investigated mechanisms that might be responsible for a reduced QoL in PCOS women. Being overweight has been found to be one of the most important contributors reducing QOL in women with PCOS [7, 22, 23]. In addition, there is converging evidence suggesting that hirsutism is one of the most important predictors of impaired QoL besides obesity [4, 23, 24]. In addition, it is demonstrated that acne, diabetes mellitus [21], menstrual irregularities [7], and concerns about infertility [4, 25, 26] are related to a reduced QoL in women with PCOS. Nevertheless, Hahn et al. [23] failed to find an association between QoL and androgens and insulin resistance.

With respect to psychological mechanisms, a reduced psychological QoL in PCOS women has been indicated to be associated with a passive coping style (a maladaptive coping strategy) [16] as well as with anxiety and depression [27].

2.2 Depression

Women with PCOS report higher levels of depressive symptoms than the general population [8]. The prevalence of depressive symptoms is not only higher but also more variable (25-64%) [12, 28-31] than for women in the general population. In addition, it has been found that women with PCOS report higher depression scores than non-PCOS controls with fertility problems [13]. PCOS features, endocrine imbalance (e.g. testosterone levels), and psychological mechanisms seem to have an impact on mood in women with PCOS and have therefore been studied as mediators of depression. For example, infertility [12] and an unfulfilled wish to conceive [27] do not appear to contribute to higher depression scores; however, infertile PCOS women seem to have higher depression scores compared to infertile women in whom infertility is related to other causes than PCOS [5]. Hence, other characteristics of PCOS seem to play a mediating role. Several studies have shown that BMI is related to depressive symptoms [22, 32, 33] as well as hirsutism and acne [11, 27]. Moreover, higher depression scores have been demonstrated in PCOS women with hirsutism compared to women with newly diagnosed gynaecological cancer [34].

PCOS is associated with high testosterone levels. Lower testosterone levels seem to be related to depression in women with PCOS [35]. Also, testosterone was found to be lower in depressive PCOS women compared to PCOS women without depressive symptoms, whereas the researchers found no significant relation between BMI and hirsutism [36]. Conversely, Barry and colleagues [13] failed to find an association between testosterone and mood disturbances in women with PCOS. Accordingly, others failed to find an association between depression and hormonal and metabolic profile [36, 37].

With respect to psychological mechanisms, it has been shown that depression in PCOS women is predicted by a poorer perception of self-worth and body image [29, 38], fitness orientation, appearance evaluation, lower QoL [29], and passive coping style (a maladaptive coping strategy) [16].

2.3 Anxiety and fears

Recently, researchers showed an increased level of anxiety [27, 29] and social anxiety [8] in PCOS women compared to controls. The finding of reduced sleep in women with PCOS might be explained by a higher prevalence of sleep apnea in obese women with PCOS [39].

An interesting issue is determining which characteristics of PCOS are related to anxiety. It has been shown that not only visual features of PCOS such as a higher body weight and an excessive growth of bodily hair were related to an increased experience of fear of what other people thought about their appearance, but also the absence of their cycle (amenorrhoea) was negatively associated with fear of appearance evaluation [40]. The association between fear of negative appearance evaluation and non-visual characteristics might be explained by a reduced feeling of femininity [10]. The experience of women with PCOS feeling less feminine seem to be related to menstrual irregularities and hirsutism [10]. Contrasting findings have been found with respect to the relation between anxiety and hirsutism. Some studies reported women with hirsutism showing greater anxiety levels [7, 11] and social fears [41]. Moreover, one study found that higher anxiety scores were indicated in PCOS women with hirsutism than in women with newly diagnosed gynaecological cancer [34]. Furthermore, both acne and an unfulfilled wish to conceive seem to be a risk factor for clinically relevant anxiety in women with PCOS [27]; however, this study failed to find a relationship for BMI and hirsutism. This is in the same line with other study results not finding a relationship between anxiety, acne, hirsutism, and BMI [36, 42]. Contrasting findings might be explained by the use of different questionnaires.

Livadas et al. [36] studied whether anxiety was associated with hormonal and metabolic profile. PCOS women with higher anxiety scores showed significantly elevated HOMA-IR (insulin resistance) and FAI (free androgen excess) values than PCOS women with lower anxiety scores, independently of BMI; however, no relation was found with hormonal values such as testosterone, androstenedione, sex hormone-binding globulin levels, dehydroepiandrosterone sulphate, and estradiol. In the same line, the relation between greater FAI values and greater levels of anxiety was previously reported by Mansson et al. [8].

Moreover, Deeks and colleagues [29] indicated in a cross-sectional study in PCOS women and controls that poor perception of self-worth and body image as well as health evaluation predicted higher anxiety levels. It has also been found that anxiety in PCOS women is associated with having a passive coping style [16].

2.4 Self-esteem and body satisfaction

A recent study demonstrated a more negative body image in women with PCOS compared to healthy controls [29]. It has been indicated that women with facial hair and decreased self-esteem have higher depression and anxiety scores as well as poorer QoL [11], although poorer self-esteem compared to the general population was not confirmed. In a previous study, we showed that women with PCOS and a higher BMI in addition to hirsutism reported having poorer self-esteem and greater body dissatisfaction than women without hirsutism and lower BMI scores. In addition, amenorrhoea was associated with poorer self-esteem whereas hyperandrogenism and acne were found to be associated with body dissatisfaction. In line with our previous findings, it has been shown that women with PCOS and clinical symptoms of hirsutism and acne have greater body dissatisfaction than healthy controls with regular cycles, even after adjustment for BMI [5, 35]. Furthermore, poorer self-esteem in PCOS women has been linked to higher levels of depression and anxiety [29, 38].

2.5 Other domains of psycho-social well-being

2.5.1 Eating disorders

A higher prevalence of eating disorders such as bulimia has been reported in women with PCOS compared to controls [8]. One study found that 12.6% of PCOS women had an eating disorder compared to 1.6% in controls [32]. No association between PCOS characteristics (such as hirsutism and acne) and eating disorders has been found [43]. Further, Livadas and colleagues [36] failed to find an association between eating disorders and hormonal and metabolic profile in women with PCOS.

2.5.2 Suicide

Mansson et al. [8] were the first who studied suicide attempts in women with PCOS: they found that suicide attempts were seven times more common in women with PCOS compared to controls [8]. This finding might be explained by the increased risk for psychological disturbances such as depression and anxiety.

2.5.3 Neuroticism and stress responses

Furthermore, a recent study reported that women with PCOS were more neurotic, meaning that they had difficulties coping with stress, exhibited more anger symptoms, and were more likely to withhold feelings of anger compared to non-PCOS women with fertility problems [44]; however, these findings disappeared with using multiple regression analyses, indicating that they might be related to distressing symptoms of the syndrome. In addition, disturbed stress responses were indicated in PCOS women [45]. This finding might be linked to the elevated risks for depression, overweight, and the cardiovascular and diabetes risks associated with the diagnosis

3. Sexual well-being in women with PCOS

Hormones play a major role in various aspects of sexuality. As PCOS is an endocrine disorder, it seems plausible that the endocrine changes associated with PCOS influence sexuality. Sexuality is an important aspect of an individual's well-being, highlighting the importance of our understanding of sexuality in women with PCOS. Existing studies with respect to PCOS and sexuality have been mainly focussing on sexual satisfaction in women with PCOS, whereas for example sexual functioning has not been given much attention. Sexual satisfaction is defined as the balance between costs and rewards concerning sexuality [46], for example: A woman without problems in the domain of sexual desire but who experiences painful intercourse has lowered sexual satisfaction because the costs (pain) are too high. Sexual functioning refers to the ability to experience the phases of the sexual response cycle (desire, arousal, lubrication, orgasm), for example: A woman who is able to feel sexually aroused but who is not able to experience an orgasm has poorer sexual functioning. Sexual satisfaction is part of sexual functioning [47] given that a person without problems in the domain of sexual functioning might experience a decreased sexual satisfaction, for example caused by negative feelings such as guilt. On the contrary, not being able to function sexual fully does not necessarily mean that one has low sexual satisfaction; one might not experience this as a problem. It is imaginable that clinicians and researchers find it more comfortable talking about sexual satisfaction than sexual functioning, with the latter being more detailed and intimate. Clinicians might not be trained in discussing sexual problems with their patients or it is unknown as to where to refer patients to with sexual problems.

3.1 Sexual functioning in women in general: The role of hormones

Androgens and estrogens play an important role in female sexual functioning. The sex steroids testosterone and estradiol play a role in all structures and organs related to female sexual functioning. For example, changes in sexual desire are noticed during changes in the menstrual cycle [48]. Sexual desire refers to a subjective feeling that is triggered by both internal and external cues, which may or may not result in overt sexual behaviour [49]. Sexual arousal has physiological and subjective aspects: the physiological part is related to an increased autonomic activation that prepares the body for sexual activity and increases the amount of sexual stimulation necessary to induce orgasm. The subjective part is related to an emotional state of arousal, including sexual thoughts and fantasies[50].

3.2 Estrogens

Estrogens play an important role in making the brain susceptible for the influence of testosterone. In addition, estrogens influence mood and physical signs of sexual attractiveness (e.g. breast development). An estrogen deficiency can cause various complaints such as mood disturbances and might indirectly influence sexuality negatively [51, 52]. It has been demonstrated in healthy pre-menopausal women without PCOS that menstrual cycle changes can influence sexual behaviour by changes in psychological well-being: improved sexual activity (frequency of partner sex, masturbation and orgasm) was related to an increased well-being (mood and pre-menstrual symptoms) [48].

Furthermore, atrophic changes (thinning of the vaginal walls) are influenced by reduced estrogen levels [53, 54]; however, sexual reactions, sexual arousal, lubrication and genital vasocongestion do not seem to be estrogen dependent. Even though estrogen levels were significantly different, studies failed to find a difference in sexual functioning between pre-menopausal and post-menopausal women [51, 52]. Likewise, no evidence has been found for a significant effect of estrogen on sexual interest, arousal, and orgasmic response [48, 53]. The best predictor for post-menopausal sexual functioning seems to pre-menopausal sexual functioning [53]. Estrogen levels are in general within the normal range in women with PCOS [55].

3.3 Androgens

Androgens have been indicated to play an important role in female sexual functioning [56] and seem to influence sexual desire and arousal (either alone or in combination with estrogen), sexual thoughts, sexual fantasies, and nocturnal genital responses [54, 57]. Androgens prepare the female sexual system to be susceptible for sexual stimuli and sexual arousal [54, 56]. Sexual arousal through non-cognitive processes (audiovisual stimulation, 'quick and dirty') has not been found to be androgen dependent, whereas sexual arousal through cognitive processes (thoughts, fantasies, 'neat and slow') has been shown to be androgen dependent [56]. Androgen levels are often increased in women with PCOS which in turn might influence sexual thoughts and desire [55]. Bancroft et al. [48] failed to find an association between testosterone levels and sexual activity with their partner; however, a positive relation was found with respect to the frequency of masturbation. Finally, testosterone and DHEAS were not found to be related with Hypoactive Sexual Desire Disorder (HSDD: a deficiency or absence of desire for sexual activity) in community based studies in women [53, 58, 59].

3.4 Hyperandrogenism and sexuality

A recent publication [60] found that not only acne and hirsutism improved by oral contraception as a result of reduced androgen levels, a positive influence on social contacts, QoL, sexual self-esteem, and feelings of sexually attractiveness has also been found. In addition, sex life in general (sexual pleasure in particular) and orgasm by intercourse improved as well as that dyspareunia (painful sexual intercourse) declined. Moreover, the frequency of intercourse increased as opposed to the frequency of masturbation. Sexual functioning seems to be improved by the mediation of improved QoL, whereas sexual self-esteem and sexual attractiveness as a result of decreasing hirsutism and acne [60]. Furthermore, Wierman and colleagues [53] found a minor influence of hyperandrogenism or its treatment on sexual functioning in women with PCOS. The researchers speculate that psycho-social factors such as decreased levels of self-esteem might have a greater impact on sexuality.

Abovementioned studies indicate that hormonal influences play a minimal role in predicting sexual functioning in women with PCOS. Lowered sexual satisfaction and sexual functioning might be mediated by psychosocial factors or by a variety in responsiveness to testosterone [61]. Finally, contextual influences (e.g. partner relationship) combined with the appropriate stimuli can cause sexual arousal resulting in sexual desire [57, 62-64].

4. Sexual functioning

4.1 Sexarche and sexual intercourse

It has been found that adolescents and women with PCOS become sexually active later in life than controls. In addition, it seems that PCOS women are less likely to have had intercourse compared to their healthy peers [7, 26, 65]. Furthermore, De Niet et al. [40] found that sexarche (the first sexual intercourse) is related to amenorrhoea; women with PCOS and amenorrhoea had an earlier sexarche than women with PCOS and oligomenorrhoea.

Although it has been indicated that PCOS women experience lower sexual satisfaction and feel less attractive than controls, the frequency of sexual intercourse [7, 66] and the number of sexual partners [66] was not found to be different compared to controls. Moreover, it has been found that the frequency of sexual intercourse increased as a result of improved QoL, sexual self-esteem, feelings of sexual attractiveness, and sexual pleasure when using oral contraceptive [60].

Pagidas et al. [67] found that intercourse compliance (2-3 times a week) was related to having an ovulatory cycle in women undergoing fertility treatment. An ovulatory cycle increased intercourse compliance, especially in women with a BMI over 35.

Painful sexual intercourse has also been studied [7, 23, 60, 66]. Two studies have found that pain during sexual intercourse is increased in women with PCOS compared to controls [23, 66]. The incidence of painful intercourse seems to be negatively influenced by BMI [23]. Painful intercourse seem to decrease with the use of oral contraceptives [60] or metformin [65], probably due to mediating factors of overall increased sexual functioning (in particular sexual pleasure).

4.2 Sexual desire

Conaglen & Conaglen [68] compared women with PCOS or idiopathic hirsutism (IH) and healthy controls on psychosocial functioning and various aspects of sexuality including sexual desire. Sexual desire was found to be significantly lower in PCOS women than in controls. After anti-androgen medication, the treatment group reported a significantly further decline in sexual desire despite a significantly increase in self-esteem and a decrease in hirsutism. This indicates that anti-androgen therapy can improve self-esteem and hirsutism, but negatively influences sexual desire. This could be due to decreasing androgen levels causing the brain to be less susceptible to sexual stimuli resulting in decreased sexual desire [54]. In line with these findings, studies failed to find a relation between sexual desire and androgen levels [57, 58, 67] in non PCOS women; however, an impaired sexual interest and desire (e.g., arousal, orgasm, pain, initiation, receptiveness, affection, relationship) was shown in with women with HSDD compared to controls [58]. In contrast, two studies indicated that women with PCOS seem to take more sexual initiative and to have greater sexual desire than controls [66, 69]. Interestingly, one study found PCOS women reporting less interest in physical contact with their partner compared to controls. These contrasting findings might be explained by psychological factors [61].

4.3 Sexual arousal, orgasm

As mentioned before, androgens influence sexual arousal; however, free or total testosterone has not been found to be related to arousal. Furthermore, it has been shown that women with PCOS are less satisfied with their sex life, had more problems with getting aroused, and showed more often no interest in physical contact with their partner compared with healthy controls [66]. In addition, insufficient lubrication was significantly higher in PCOS women [11]. This finding seems to explain the higher incidence of painful sexual intercourse.

The incidence of sexual thoughts and fantasies (part of subjective arousal) seems to be negatively correlated to BMI [23]; however, orgasm frequency was not found to differ between PCOS women and controls [66]. In addition, total serum testosterone but not FAI was positively related to higher scores in aspects of sexual functioning (such as satisfaction sex life, frequency of orgasm during intercourse, and vaginal lubrication) in PCOS women [66]. A hypothesis is that levels of testosterone above average improve sexual functioning; however, this is not in line with other findings [12, 23, 66, 68].

Using oral contraceptives seem to improve the frequency of orgasm during intercourse in women with PCOS [60], probably due to mediating factors as improved sexual pleasure, sexual self-esteem, and BMI. One study [70] failed to find a difference in sexual functioning or in genital anatomy between lean PCOS women and lean controls. Despite differences in androgen levels, no difference was found in clitoral volume and vascularisation.

4.4 Sexual satisfaction, attractiveness, and self-worth

It is widely recognized that women with PCOS report a decreased sexual satisfaction than healthy controls [7, 12, 26, 65, 66]. Sexual satisfaction seems to be influenced by both endocrine and psycho-social factors. For example, both BMI and hirsutism seem to negatively influence sexual satisfaction, sexual attractiveness [23], and body esteem [68]. PCOS women also thought that their partners found them less sexually attractive [12]. Using an oral contraceptive improved hirsutism and acne [60, 68] which led to an improved feeling of sexual attractiveness and sexual self-esteem [60].

Sexual self-worth seems to be lower in PCOS women [12, 17]. This finding might be related to infertility; however, this association could not be established. No other studies were found using the term self-worth. Self-esteem was reported [60, 68] and seem to be related to hirsutism and acne [68, 71].

Furthermore, it seems that BMI, hirsutism, and acne negatively influence making social contacts [12, 23] in women with PCOS. This finding might be explained by lower levels of self-esteem and other psychosocial factors [70].

Finally, poorer body-image has been found to be associated with sexual avoidance [38] in women with PCOS compared to controls. Likewise, depression as a consequence of BMI was also found to have a negative association with sexual functioning in pre-menopausal women [72]. A similar relation might be expected in women with PCOS. In the same line, psychosocial aspects seem to negatively influence sexuality in women with PCOS: impaired psychological well-being [7, 60, 68], partner relationship [47], general health [65], social influences [59], and quality of the sexual stimuli [47].

4.5 Sex-typed behaviour and sexual orientation in PCOS women

Last, there is evidence that sex typed behaviour and sexual orientations are related to hormonal levels. One study measured sex-typed behaviour online as well as self-reported PCOS diagnosis [73]. The results indicated that PCOS women reported significantly less typical feminine behaviour as a child (e.g., experimenting with make-up). In addition, PCOS women reported to have lower rates of dating boys and being part of a sports team.

The results of studies examining the prevalence of PCOS in lesbian women and heterosexual women are contrasting. For example, Smith et al. [74] did not find a difference in the prevalence of PCOS and associated factors (e.g. hirsutism and testosterone level) in a general population of lesbian and heterosexual women. In contrast, another study conducted in a clinical population found a significant higher prevalence of PCOS and associated factors in lesbian than in heterosexual women [75].

Finally, one study found that higher testosterone levels and a higher incidence of hirsutism, acne, menstrual irregularities as well as a higher prevalence of PCOS in female-to-male transsexuals (FMT) [76].

5. Part II

The objective of Part II was to evaluate the association between PCOS characteristics (polycystic ovaries, hirsutism, acne, menstrual irregularities (amenorrhea and oligomenorrhea), and BMI) and endocrine variables (e.g., testosterone and estradiol) on the one hand and sexual well-being on the other hand. In addition, we studied whether there is an association between aspects of psycho-social well-being (self-esteem, body satisfaction, and self-perceived fear of negative appearance evaluation) and sexual well-being.

6. Methods

6.1 Participants and procedure

Women with normogonadotropic anovulation (WHO II) who attended our fertility clinic at the Erasmus MC University Medical Centre between 1991 and 2006 were included in this cross-sectional study. In this group of WHO II women, we determined if the diagnosis of PCOS could be established on the basis of the revised Rotterdam criteria [77]. To establish the diagnosis of PCOS, all patients underwent a standardized evaluation including: assessing cycle history, the presence or absence of acne, transvaginal ultrasonography (to assess ovarian volume and follicle count for both ovaries), and anthropomorphometric measurements (height and weight, Ferriman-Gallwey score). Exclusion criteria included the presence of related disorders with similar clinical presentation, such as congenital adrenal hyperplasia and Cushing's syndrome. The study protocol was approved by the Medical Ethics Committee of the Erasmus MC University Medical Centre, Rotterdam the Netherlands. All patients gave informed consent prior to their inclusion in the present study. In 2007, all women with WHO II received a letter with information about the current study and a seventy-two item questionnaire. Two months after mailing this questionnaire, non-respondents were sent a reminder together with a copy of the questionnaire.

6.2 Study outcomes

6.2.1 Independent variables: PCOS characteristics and endocrine variables

In the period of 1991 to 2006, all women who were referred to the fertility clinic underwent a standard fertility test including evaluation of the following aspects:

1. Menstrual irregularities: oligomenorrhoea was defined as an interval between menstrual periods ≥35 days and amenorrhoea as the absence of vaginal bleeding for at least 6 months, i.e. >199 days;
2. Biochemical and clinical hyperandrogenism: in accordance with the revised Rotterdam criteria, hyperandrogenism was defined as having either biochemical or clinical signs of androgen excess. Biochemical hyperandrogenism was defined by a free androgen index (FAI)>4.5. Clinical hyperandrogenism (hirsutism) was assessed by the Ferriman-Gallwey score where patients estimated their hair growth on nine different body parts from 0 (no terminal hair) to 4 (maximal growth) with a maximum score of 36. A score of 8 or more indicates the presence of hirsutism [78];
3. Acne: the presence or absence of acne was evaluated by the physician;
4. Polycystic ovaries (PCO): the presence of PCO was examined by vaginal ultrasound examination. PCO were defined as the presence of 12 follicles or more in one or both ovaries and/or increased ovarian volume (>10 ml); and
5. Endocrine evaluation: blood samples were obtained by venipuncture. Serum levels of gonadotropic hormones (luteinizing hormone (LH) and follicle-stimulating hormone (FSH)), estradiol (E_2), androgens (testosterone (T), androstenedione (AD), dehydroepiandrosterone (DHEA), and dehydroepiandrosterone sulphate (DHEAS)), progesterone, sex hormone-binding globulin levels (SHBG), fasting glucose and insulin, thyroid-stimulating hormone (TSH), and prolactin were obtained. Serum was isolated after centrifugation at 3000 rpm for 10 min at 20°C and subsequently stored at -20°C.

Immunofluorometric assays were used for the LH, FSH, TSH, prolactin and insulin, whereas serum E_2, T, AD, and SHBG were measured by RIA provided by Diagnostic Products Corp. (Los Angelas, CA). Intraassay and interassay coefficients of variation were <5% and <15% for LH, <3% and <5% for T, <8% and <11% for AD, <5% and <7% for E_2, <4% and <5% for SHBG, respectively [3].

6.2.2 Independent variables: Psycho-social well-being

6.2.2.1 Rosenberg Self-Esteem Scale (RSES)

The RSES was administered to measure the level of self-esteem. On a 4-point-Likert scale from 'strongly disagree' to 'strongly agree', responses on 5 positively worded and 5 negatively worded questions were assessed. Higher scores reflect a higher level of self-esteem. The Dutch version of the RSES was shown to have good internal reliability (Chronbach's alpha = .87) [79].

6.2.2.2 Body Cathexis Scale (BCS)

The BCS is a self-report questionnaire assessing body satisfaction [80]. The questionnaire consists of 52 items about a person's satisfaction with their body parts and body functions, such as hips and respiration. Body satisfaction is measured on a 5-point Likert scale from the most negative attitude towards a body part or function to the most positive attitude towards the body part or function. The Dutch version of the questionnaire was shown to have good test-retest reliability (Pearson product-moment correlation coefficient = .91) [81].

6.2.2.3 Fear of Negative Appearance Evaluation Scale (FNAES)

The brief version of the FNAES was used to assess apprehension related to a negative appearance evaluative experience. The items are answered on 5-point Likert scales from 'not at all' to 'enormously'. The higher the score, the more fear of negative appearance evaluation by others is experienced. This six-item questionnaire was shown to be valid and reliable with a high internal consistency (Chronbach's α=0.87) [82]

6.2.3 Dependent variables: Sexual well-being

6.2.3.1 Sexual well-being

Subjects completed questions that were part of a Dutch questionnaire measuring sexual health in youth and young adults between the age of 12 and 25 years [83]. The questions that we used in the current study included the following: (1) *'How old were you when you had your first intercourse?'*; (2) *'Have you ever had a romantic relationship?'*; (3) *'How old were you when you had your first romantic relationship?'*; (4) *'Have you ever been in love?'*; and (5) *Are you in a romantic relationship at this moment?'*

6.2.3.2 Confounders: Demographics

Information on women's demographic characteristics such as age and ethnicity were collected. Ethnicity was divided into two categories: (0) non-Caucasian (another ethnicity than Dutch) and (1) Caucasian (Dutch).

7. Statistical analyses

Data are presented for women with PCOS only. As measures for central tendency the means (for continuous data) and medians (for ordinal data) were estimated, while as measure for dispersion standard deviation was used. The observed score range was also presented. To explore the association between sexual well-being variables (dependent variables) on the one hand and the PCOS characteristics and endocrine variables or psycho-social well-being (independent variables) on the other hand, multiple linear regression analysis was applied on continuous dependent variables. The PCOS characteristics and endocrine variables were entered into the regression analysis together with confounding variables (age and ethnicity). Psychological variables were analyzed separately. For dichotomous dependent variables, adjusted odds ratios (Ors) and 99% confidence intervals (CI) were derived from logistic regression analyses. PCOS characteristics were entered as dichotomous variables: oligoamenorrhoea (0) versus amenorrhoea (1); no or doubtful hirsutism (0) versus hirsutism (1); few or no acne (0) versus acne (1); no PCO (0) versus PCO (1). In analyzing the relationship between sexuality and PCOS characteristics, we adjusted for the time interval between the date of the clinical evaluation and the sexuality measures, age of the participant, and ethnicity. As sexarche was prior to the clinical investigation for most women, we entered years between sexarche and the clinical evaluation as a confounding variable in the analyses. Ethnicity was entered as a confounding variable because non-Caucasian women appeared to have sexarche later in life and higher clinical scores such as hirsutism than Caucasian women. Statistical analyses were performed using the Statistical Package for the Social Sciences (SPSS version 15.0) and testing took place at a 0.05 level of significance (two tailed).

8. Imputation

Multiple imputation was performed using the SPSS software in the Missing Value Analysis module in SPSS (version 17.0) to impute missing values under missing-at-random assumptions and the reasons for the missing data are unrelated to the outcome [84]. Multiple imputed data sets of the data were created and replaced by imputed values based on estimated underlying distributions using the Expectation Maximization method [85]. Eight variables were imputed, of which six variables had ≤ than 1.5% imputed data. The variable acne (68%) and hirsutism (35%) had a high percentage of imputed data, numbers of missings that are controversy to impute.

9. Results

9.1 Participants

In the period between 1991 and 2006, 1148 WHO II patients attended the fertility clinic of the Erasmus MC University Medical Centre and underwent standard clinical and endocrine evaluation. Of the 1148 women with WHO II, 480 women with PCOS returned the questionnaire. The overall participation rate was 51% of whom 42% had PCOS. Table I shows the demographical, clinical, endocrine, psychological, and sexual characteristics of the responders with PCOS in our study. It has been indicated that a higher percentage of non-responders with PCOS were overweight or obese and had hyperandrogenism compared to the responders [40]. In addition, we showed that PCOS women had lower self-esteem and poorer body satisfaction compared to norm scores. Of the women that completed the sexuality questions, 2.1% responded that they had their first sexual intercourse when they were of the age of 13 years or younger and 4.0% had their first relationship when they were13 years or younger.

	PCOS responders (n=480)
Demographical characteristics	
Age in years at date of clinical evaluation	28.8 (4.3), 14.2-40.0 (480)
Caucasian	72.1% (346/480)
Clinical	
Oligoamenorrhoea	71.7% (344/480)
Amenorrea	28.3% (136/480)
Presence of hirsutism	31.9% (99/310)
Acne	11% (17/154)
PCO	92.5% (444/480)
Body Mass Index (BMI kg/m²)	26.4 (6.0) [16.8-50.6] (479)
BMI ≥ 25 (kg/m²)	48.6% (233/479)
Endocrine	
Hyperandrogenism (FAI>4.5)	53.1% (255/480)
LH	7.2 (5.6) [1.0-37.9] (480)
FSH	4.9 (1.9) [1.1-10.5] (480)
Progesterone	5.1 (10.1) [0.1 - 73.0] (479)
SHBG	49.2 (33.3) [7.7 - 342] (480)
T	2.2 (1.0) [0.3 - 6.7] (480)
E_2	275.8 (159.9) [51.0 - 1141.0]
AD	13.0 (5.7) [2.6 - 40.7]
DHEAS	6.0 (3.2) [0.2 - 21.3]
Psycho-social well-being	
RSES	31.0 (5.4) [14.0-40.0] (477)
BCS	188.6 (30.3) [72.0 - 260.0] (435)
FNAES	13.8 (5.9) [6.0 - 30.0] (473)
Sexual well-being	
'Are you in a romantic relationship at this moment?' %yes	92.7% (443/478)
'Have you ever been in love?'	
% Never or 1 time	14.4% (69/473)
% More than 1 time	84.2% (404/473)
'Have you ever had a romantic relationship?'	
% Never or 1 time	41.6% (198/478)
% More than 1 time	58.3% (280/478)
'How old were you when you had your first intercourse?'	18.4 (3.3) [5.0 - 30.0] (467)
'How old were you when you had your first romantic relationship?'	17.7 (3.2) [10.0 - 30.0] (471)

PCO= Polycystic ovaries; LH= luteinizing hormone; FSH= follicle-stimulating hormone; SHBG= sex hormone-binding globulin levels; DHEAS= dehydroepiandrosterone sulphate; T= Testosterone; E_2= Estradiol; AD= Androstenedione; RSES= Rosenberg Self-esteem Scale; BCS= Body Cathexis Scale; FNAES= Fear of Negative Appearance Evaluation Scale.

[1]Values are mean (SD), range, N or (N/total N), or number (%) of participants.

Table 1. Demographical and (bio)clinical characteristics of PCOS responders[1]

9.2 PCOS characteristics and endocrine variables and the association with sexual well-being

Table II shows the regression coefficients (B's) and corresponding P-values derived by the logistic and linear multivariate regression analyses studying the association between the dependent sexual well-being variables and independent PCOS symptoms and endocrine variables.

Relationship at the moment

Results indicated that oligomenorrhoea was positively associated with having a relationship at the moment. In addition, the confounder ethnicity was also significant. These results indicated that PCOS women with oligomenorrhoea were more likely than women with amenorrhea to have a relationship at the moment. In addition, Caucasian PCOS women were more likely to have a relationship at the time of questionnaire completion than non-Caucasian PCOS women.

In love

Older PCOS women, Caucasian women, and women without or doubtful hirsutism were more likely to have been in love multiple times as compared to younger PCOS women.

Relationship in the past

The results showed that the confounders ethnicity, age, and the years between measuring the clinical/endocrine variables and sexuality variables were significant in logistic analysis: Caucasian women and older women were more likely to have had more than one relationship in the past.

Age at first intercourse

Non-Caucasian women and older women have had their first intercourse at an older age than younger and Caucasian PCOS women.

Age at first relationship

With respect to the age of the first relationship, we found women with PCOS and hirsutism and older women with PCOS were comparatively older when they had their first relationship. In addition, non-Caucasian women had their first relationship at an older age compared to Caucasian women.

		DEPENDENT	VARIABLES			
	Relationship at the moment	In love	Relationship in the past		Age first intercourse	Age first relationship
Logistic regression	B; P-value; odds	B; P-value; odds	B; P-value; odds	*Multivariate regression*	B; P-value	B; P-value
PCO	-1.33; 0.44 0.26	0.85; 0.55; 2.33	-0.12; 0.81; 0.89		-0.00; 1.00	-0.02; 0.97
Cycle disturbances	-0.99; **0.04***; 0.37	-0.24; 0.49; 0.79	-0.24; 0.30; 0.79		-0.26; 0.45	-0.12; 0.72
Acné	2.01; 1.00; 7.48	4.69; 1.00; 108.83	-0.52; 0.42; 0.59		0.21; 0.75	0.38; 0.53

	DEPENDENT VARIABLES					
	Relationship at the moment	In love	Relationship in the past		Age first intercourse	Age first relationship
Hirsutism	-0.94; 0.10; 0.39	-1.17; **0.009***; 0.31	-0.43; 0.14; 0.65		0.79; 0.07	1.29; **0.002***
BMI	0.07; 0.16; 1.07	0.01; 0.79; 1.01	0.00; 0.82; 1.00		-0.04; 0.12	-0.04; 0.17
T	0.30; 0.40; 1.35	0.20; 0.38; 1.22	0.22; 0.15; 1.25		0.02; 0.94	-0.16; 0.44
E2	0.00; 0.59; 1.00	0.00; 0.81; 1.00	0.00; 0.19; 1.00		0.00; 0.38	-0.00; 0.13
Progesterone	-0.02; 0.43; 0.98	-0.01; 0.45; 0.99	-0.01; 0.32; 0.99		0.02; 0.33	0.02; 0.14
AD	0.08; 0.24; 1.09	0.03; 0.48; 1.03	0.04; 0.13; 1.04		0.00; 0.97	-0.02; 0.61
SHBG	0.01; 0.26; 1.01	-0.00; 0.77; 1.00	0.00; 0.92; 1.00		0.00; 0.68	0.01; 0.13
DHEAS	-0.07; 0.39; 0.93	0.02; 0.73; 1.02	0.01; 0.79; 1.01		0.03; 0.64	0.04; 0.48
Age	0.08; 0.12; 1.08	0.10; **0.01***; 1.10	0.08; **0.003***; 1.08		0.17; **0.000***	0.12; **0.001***
Yrs between sexarche and clinical evaluation					-0.12; 0.07	
Ethnicity	-1.35; **0.008***; 0.23	-1.13; **0.001***; 0.32	-0.56; **0.02***; 0.57		1.73; **0.000***	1.56; **0.000***
Yrs between sexual variables and clinical evaluation	0.00; 1.00; 1.00	-0.23; **0.001***; 0.79	-0.16; **0.000***; 0.85			-0.14; **0.027***

PCO= Polycystic ovaries; BMI= Body Mass Index; T= Testosterone; E2= Estradiol; AD= Androstenedione; SHBG= sex hormone-binding globulin levels; DHEAS= dehydroepiandrosterone sulphate.
*Significant at a 0.05 level of significance

Table 2. The association between the dependent sexual well-being variables and independent PCOS symptoms and endocrine variables

9.3 Psycho-social well-being and the association with sexual well-being

Table III shows the regression coefficients (B's) with corresponding P-values derived by the logistic and linear multivariate regression analyses analyzing the association between the dependent sexual well-being variables and independent psycho-social well-being variables.

Relationship at the moment

In logistic regression analysis studying the association between having a relationship at the moment and psycho-social variables, we found that older PCOS women and Caucasian women were more likely to have a relationship at the moment than younger and non-Caucasian PCOS women.

In love

PCOS women with higher self-esteem and Caucasian women were more likely to have been in love multiple times.

Relationship in the past

Being Caucasian, having higher self-esteem and lower body satisfaction scores were associated with having had multiples relationship in the past.

Age at first intercourse

Being older and non-Caucasian were both associated with having experienced the first intercourse at an older age.

Age at first relationship

Finally, PCOS women with lower levels of self-esteem as well as women with greater body satisfaction had their first relationship at an older age. Also, both older women with PCOS and non-Caucasian PCOS women were more likely to be comparatively older when they had their first relationship.

		DEPENDENT	VARIABLES			
	Relationship at the moment	In love	Relationship in the past		Age first intercourse	Age first relationship
Logistic regression	B; P-value; odds	B; P-value; odds	B; P-value; odds	***Multivariate regression***	B; P-value;	B; P-value;
RSES	0.08; 0.07; 1.08	0.10; **0.003***; 1.10	0.06; **0.02***; 1.01		-0.06; 0.15	-0.09; **0.02***
BCS	-0.01; 0.30; 0.99	-0.01; 0.11; 0.99	-0.01; **0.04***; 1.00		0.01; 0.17	0.02; **0.01***
FNAES	-0.01; 0.84; 0.99	0.05; 0.09; 1.05	0.03; 0.22; 1.03		-0.02; 0.60	0.00; 0.97
Age	0.08; **0.02***; 1.08	0.01; 0.76; 1.01	0.01; 0.51; 1.01		0.12; **0.000***	0.08; **0.004***
Ethnicity	-1.13; **0.002***; 0.32	-1.21; **0.000***; 0.30	-0.53; **0.01***; 0.59		1.75; **0.000***	1.57; **0.000***

RSES= Rosenberg Self-esteem Scale; BCS= Body Cathexis Scale; FNAES= Fear of Negative Appearance Evaluation Scale.
*Significant at a 0.05 level of significance

Table 3. The association between the dependent sexual well-being variables and independent psycho-social well-being variables

10. Discussion

A higher incidence of psycho-social disturbances [8] and impaired sexual well-being [7, 26, 65] in women with PCOS highlight the clinical relevance of these topics. To improve overall well-being in women with PCOS, we need to have a better understanding to what extent the features of the syndrome affect psycho-social and sexual well-being.

The current study examined the association of PCOS characteristics and endocrine variables with sexual well-being. In addition, we studied whether psycho-social well-being was associated with sexual health. First, we found that several PCOS characteristics and endocrine parameters predicted sexual well-being. PCOS women with amenorrhoea seem to be less likely to have had a relationship at the time of completing the questionnaire. It is imaginable that an irregular cycle causes distress in women, which might have withheld them from starting a romantic relationship. In the same line, it has been found that menstrual irregularities decrease QoL [7] and are linked to fear of negative appearance evaluation [40]. An association between menstrual irregularities and any aspect of sexual health has not been confirmed previously [7].

Furthermore, we found that women with PCOS and hirsutism were less likely to have been in love more than once and were older when they had their first relationship. It is widely recognized that hirsutism is one of the many factors that has a considerable negative impact on QoL [21], self-esteem, body satisfaction [5, 35, 40], and sexual health [23]. Hirsutism is considered as one of the most stressful characteristics of PCOS [10]. As women with PCOS and hirsutism also experience greater fear of negative appearance evaluation [40] and excessive body hair seem to withhold PCOS women from making social contacts [7], it seems plausible to assume that this negatively affects starting a romantic relationship.

With respect to the studied endocrine variables, we did not find that hormonal and endocrine variables are associated with sexual health. In contrast, other studies showed that higher levels of T and androgens are associated with higher levels of sexual arousal and sexual desire [54, 66, 86], although an association with DHEAS was not confirmed in a previous study [58]. However, we measured different aspects of sexual well-being. Other studies showed decreased lubrication [66], lower levels of arousal, and improvement of orgasm frequency by using oral contraceptives [60]. Furthermore, lower levels of T seem to be associated with depression [42], which might also have indirectly influenced sexual well-being. Contrasting results have been found with respect to sexual desire in PCOS women [66, 69, 87]. Anti-androgen therapy seems to further lower sexual desire, even though it improved psychological well-being [68]. Contrasting results with respect to the association between androgens and sexual desire [66, 69, 87] indicate that androgen levels are as yet unreliable predictors of sexual functioning, specifically for sexual desire. It is hypothesized that contradicting findings concerning the role of androgens in female sexual functioning may be due to, among other factors, a greater variety in responsiveness to testosterone in women and mediation of psychological mechanisms [61].

With respect to the significant result of the confounder age, it is imaginable that older women have different norms and values concerning sexuality and romantic relationships. For example, it is not inconceivable that the age of having first sexual intercourse or a relationship is younger in the present time than in previous generations. In addition, the confounder ethnicity is also associated with sexual well-being. Possible differences in sexual morality and cultural backgrounds might have caused non-Caucasian women to have their first intercourse at an older age.

Surprisingly, BMI and acne were not found to predict any of our measured sexual well-being variables. We might have failed to find an effect for acne since this variable had much missing data. Imputing high percentages of missing data is controversial; however, when we analyzed the data again on non-imputed data. The results still indicated a non-significant effect of acne. Also, Progesterone, SHBG, and E_2 were not related to sexual health in the current study.

Second, we studied the association between psycho-social variables and sexual health. Women with PCOS seem to have poorer self-esteem and poorer body satisfaction compared to the general population [40]. In addition, it is indicated that PCOS characteristics such as hirsutism, menstrual irregularities, and BMI are related to impaired psychological functioning [40]. In the current study, we demonstrated that self-esteem plays a significant role in sexual health. We showed that PCOS women with greater self-esteem are more likely have been in love multiple times, to have had more than one relationship in the past, and to have their first relationship at a younger age compared to PCOS women with poorer self-esteem. Decreased sexual satisfaction has been reported in PCOS women [7, 26, 65, 66], which is negatively correlated to BMI and hirsutism. Improving hirsutism and acne, for instance by using an oral contraceptive, seem to improve sexual satisfaction, sexual attractiveness, and self-esteem [60, 68, 71]. Furthermore, an improvement in QoL seems to be related to an increase in the frequency of sexual intercourse and satisfaction with sex life in women with PCOS [7, 65]. Also, it has been shown that BMI, hirsutism, acne negatively influences making social contacts in women with PCOS [61], probably due to low self-esteem. Therefore, it seems conceivable that women with higher levels of self-esteem feel more confident to make social contact and specifically start romantic relationships. Surprisingly, we found that women with greater body satisfaction were older when they had their first relationship. Likewise, it is indicated that body dissatisfaction increased the probability of coitus onset in adolescent girls [88]. Future research should further investigate this relationship. Fear of negative appearance evaluation was not related to any of the sexual variables. This is surprising as it would be plausible to assume that if a person fears what others think of their appearance, they are less likely to be involved in romantic relationships. A recent study indicated that increased anxiety predicted lifelong female sexual dysfunctioning in a sample of the general population [89]. Future research should focus on the relation of anxiety and sexual health in women with PCOS.

Pitfalls of studies conducting research on psycho-social and sexual well-being in women with PCOS include the use of self-reported measures. Self-reported questionnaires measure mostly mental symptoms but not clinical syndromes. Mansson et al. [8] did use clinical structured interviews to assess DSM-IV diagnoses and did show psychiatric disorders such as depression and anxiety to be more common in women with PCOS compared to controls. Other drawbacks of our study include that the PCOS women completed the questionnaires later in time than the laboratory and clinical tests were performed. Patients reasonably would have scored the psychological questionnaires different at the time when laboratory and clinical parameters were measured and reported to them. Therefore, we also adjusted for the time interval in years between the endocrine evaluation and the psychological measures. Furthermore, we did not include a matched control group. The current results therefore particularly apply to differences within the PCOS population. Finally, the non-responding rate in our study was high [40]. This might be due to a high percentage of non-Caucasian patients in the non-responding group. A possible explanation is that the Caucasian non-responders had trouble filling out the questionnaires due to insufficient command of the Dutch language. Therefore the results could not be generalized to all women with PCOS. Furthermore, it might be that those women returning the questionnaire were those PCOS women whose psycho-social and sexual well-being were the least affected by their syndrome. In the latter case, the impact of PCOS on psycho-social and sexual well-being might even be underestimated. The impact of symptoms of PCOS on sexual well-being established in the current study might also be underestimated because the non-responders harboured the more pronounced phenotypes.

In conclusion, this study stresses that the treatment of women with PCOS should notably focus not only on physical but also on psycho-social and sexual well-being. Future research should study various aspects of sexuality, e.g. sexual satisfaction, sexual motivation, and sexual self-esteem in randomized control trials with validated questionnaires as well as the influence of PCOS features. To fully understand the correlation between PCOS and sexuality, future studies should take all confounders (endocrine, psychological, and interpersonal) into account.

11. Clinical management

The overview provided in this chapter demonstrates the considerable impact of PCOS and its symptoms on psycho-social and sexual health. As women with PCOS are four times more likely to have abnormal depression scores compared to controls [90] This risk was independent of BMI, therefore it seems necessary to screen all women with PCOS for depression using validated measurements. Moreover, the literature shows an impairment of a variety of psycho-social and sexual health domains in women with PCOS and associations with features of PCOS characteristics. Therefore, we recommend assessing psycho-social and sexual domains by validated measurements.

An important finding is that treatment of associated PCOS characteristics seems to improve psychological and sexual outcomes. For example, metformin or oral contraceptive pill treatment in women with PCOS seems to be related to a reduction of clinical symptoms as well as to an improved psychological and sexual well-being [65]. In addition, using an oral contraceptive [60] or metformin [65] seems to decrease the frequency of painful intercourse. A reduction in body weight and normalized menstrual cycle seems to have mediated these findings. Various oral contraceptives seem to have a different effect on sexuality and psychosocial factors [60, 68, 91]. This should be taken into account when prescribing these medications.

Furthermore, the presence of obesity in PCOS women is associated with various physical consequences and psychological impairments. Lifestyle modification should be the first step before treating PCOS women for their infertility. Various studies have investigated the effects of weight loss and weight loss interventions in women with PCOS, indicating the beneficial effects of weight loss on the clinical and biochemical manifestations of PCOS [92, 93], insulin sensitivity [94], and menstrual cyclicality and fertility outcomes during treatment [95, 96]. Moreover, self-esteem [95] and quality of life [97] have found to be improved by modest weight loss of 5% to 10% of the initial body weight. We also discussed the considerable impact of hirsutism on several psychosocial and sexual domains. It has been shown that laser treatment aimed at reducing the severity of facial hirsutism has not only a positive effect on the severity of facial hair, but also seems to improve self-esteem and QoL [98] and alleviate depression and anxiety [99]. Therefore, treatment of related PCOS symptoms should be considered.

A recent paper of Farrell and colleagues [37] demonstrated the benefits of psychological and behavioural approaches in addition to medical management of PCOS. Likewise, Rofey et al. [38] found decreased depression scores as well as weight loss after a behavioural program in adolescents with PCOS. The intervention consisted of phone calls and face to face meetings addressing coping mechanisms, scheduling behaviourally activating events, and engaging in positive thinking and cognitive restructuring. Furthermore, another study showed that a nurse-led peer support group providing socio-emotional and informational support reduced isolation and women reported feeling empowered [100].

Bitzer et al. [101] developed a tool for sexual counselling that can be used by physicians. It contains 3 dimensions (pre-existing person related factors, disease specific factors, and the individual's and partners reaction to the disease) that can be addressed when discussing sexuality with the patient. Remembering these dimensions is fairly easy and gives a good direction in discussing sexuality aspects with patients. A treatment plan might depend on the outcome of the conversation. Another easy-to-use tool is the PLISSIT model [102]. This is a stepped care model providing guidance in counselling and treating sexual problems.

Aforementioned treatments and their positive effect on psycho-social and sexual well-being indicate that physicians should work interdisciplinary to also address consequences other than physical consequences and discuss treatment options aimed at reducing PCOS characteristics and improving psycho-social and sexual well-being.

12. References

[1] Ehrmann DA, Liljenquist DR, Kasza K, Azziz R, Legro RS, Ghazzi MN. Prevalence and predictors of the metabolic syndrome in women with polycystic ovary syndrome. J Clin Endocrinol Metab. 2006 Jan;91(1):48-53.

[2] Laven JS, Imani B, Eijkemans MJ, Fauser BC. New approach to polycystic ovary syndrome and other forms of anovulatory infertility. Obstet Gynecol Surv. 2002 Nov;57(11):755-67.

[3] Valkenburg O, Steegers-Theunissen RP, Smedts HP, Dallinga-Thie GM, Fauser BC, Westerveld EH, et al. A more atherogenic serum lipoprotein profile is present in women with polycystic ovary syndrome: a case-control study. J Clin Endocrinol Metab. 2008 Feb;93(2):470-6.

[4] Elsenbruch S, Benson S, Hahn S, Tan S, Mann K, Pleger K, et al. Determinants of emotional distress in women with polycystic ovary syndrome. Hum Reprod. 2006 Apr;21(4):1092-9.

[5] Himelein MJ, Thatcher SS. Depression and body image among women with polycystic ovary syndrome. J Health Psychol. 2006 Jul;11(4):613-25.

[6] Himelein MJ, Thatcher SS. Polycystic ovary syndrome and mental health: A review. Obstet Gynecol Surv. 2006 Nov;61(11):723-32.

[7] Elsenbruch S, Hahn S, Kowalsky D, Offner AH, Schedlowski M, Mann K, et al. Quality of life, psychosocial well-being, and sexual satisfaction in women with polycystic ovary syndrome. J Clin Endocrinol Metab. 2003 Dec;88(12):5801-7.

[8] Mansson M, Holte J, Landin-Wilhelmsen K, Dahlgren E, Johansson A, Landen M. Women with polycystic ovary syndrome are often depressed or anxious--a case control study. Psychoneuroendocrinology. 2008 Sep;33(8):1132-8.

[9] Sills ES, Perloe M, Tucker MJ, Kaplan CR, Genton MG, Schattman GL. Diagnostic and treatment characteristics of polycystic ovary syndrome: descriptive measurements of patient perception and awareness from 657 confidential self-reports. BMC women's health. 2001;1(1):3.
[10] Kitzinger C, Willmott J. 'The thief of womanhood': women's experience of polycystic ovarian syndrome. Soc Sci Med. 2002 Feb;54(3):349-61.
[11] Lipton MG, Sherr L, Elford J, Rustin MH, Clayton WJ. Women living with facial hair: the psychological and behavioral burden. J Psychosom Res. 2006 Aug;61(2):161-8.
[12] Tan S, Hahn S, Benson S, Janssen OE, Dietz T, Kimmig R, et al. Psychological implications of infertility in women with polycystic ovary syndrome. Hum Reprod. 2008 Sep;23(9):2064-71.
[13] Barry JA, Bouloux P, Hardiman PJ. The impact of eating behavior on psychological symptoms typical of reactive hypoglycemia. A pilot study comparing women with polycystic ovary syndrome to controls. Appetite. 2011 Mar 21;57(1):73-6.
[14] Cattrall FR, Healy DL. Long-term metabolic, cardiovascular and neoplastic risks with polycystic ovary syndrome. Best Pract Res Clin Obstet Gynaecol. 2004 Oct;18(5):803-12.
[15] Hardiman P, Pillay OC, Atiomo W. Polycystic ovary syndrome and endometrial carcinoma. Lancet. 2003 May 24;361(9371):1810-2.
[16] Benson S, Hahn S, Tan S, Janssen OE, Schedlowski M, Elsenbruch S. Maladaptive coping with illness in women with polycystic ovary syndrome. J Obstet Gynecol Neonatal Nurs. 2010 Jan;39(1):37-45.
[17] Janssen OE, Hahn S, Tan S, Benson S, Elsenbruch S. Mood and sexual function in polycystic ovary syndrome. Semin Reprod Med. 2008 Jan;26(1):45-52.
[18] Jones GL, Hall JM, Balen AH, Ledger WL. Health-related quality of life measurement in women with polycystic ovary syndrome: a systematic review. Hum Reprod Update. 2008 Jan-Feb;14(1):15-25.
[19] Coffey S, Bano G, Mason HD. Health-related quality of life in women with polycystic ovary syndrome: a comparison with the general population using the Polycystic Ovary Syndrome Questionnaire (PCOSQ) and the Short Form-36 (SF-36). Gynecol Endocrinol. 2006 Feb;22(2):80-6.
[20] Cronin L, Guyatt G, Griffith L, Wong E, Azziz R, Futterweit W, et al. Development of a health-related quality-of-life questionnaire (PCOSQ) for women with polycystic ovary syndrome (PCOS). J Clin Endocrinol Metab. 1998 Jun;83(6):1976-87.
[21] Coffey S, Mason H. The effect of polycystic ovary syndrome on health-related quality of life. Gynecol Endocrinol. 2003 Oct;17(5):379-86.
[22] Barnard L, Ferriday D, Guenther N, Strauss B, Balen AH, Dye L. Quality of life and psychological well being in polycystic ovary syndrome. Hum Reprod. 2007 Aug;22(8):2279-86.
[23] Hahn S, Janssen OE, Tan S, Pleger K, Mann K, Schedlowski M, et al. Clinical and psychological correlates of quality-of-life in polycystic ovary syndrome. Eur J Endocrinol. 2005 Dec;153(6):853-60.
[24] Trent M, Austin SB, Rich M, Gordon CM. Overweight status of adolescent girls with polycystic ovary syndrome: body mass index as mediator of quality of life. Ambul Pediatr. 2005 Mar-Apr;5(2):107-11.

[25] Pekhlivanov B, Kolarov G, Kavurdzhikova S, Stoikov S. [Determinants of health related quality of life in women with polycystic ovary syndrome]. Akush Ginekol (Sofiia). 2006;45(7):29-34.

[26] Trent ME, Rich M, Austin SB, Gordon CM. Fertility concerns and sexual behavior in adolescent girls with polycystic ovary syndrome: implications for quality of life. J Pediatr Adolesc Gynecol. 2003 Feb;16(1):33-7.

[27] Benson S, Hahn S, Tan S, Mann K, Janssen OE, Schedlowski M, et al. Prevalence and implications of anxiety in polycystic ovary syndrome: results of an internet-based survey in Germany. Hum Reprod. 2009 Jun;24(6):1446-51.

[28] Bhattacharya SM, Jha A. Prevalence and risk of depressive disorders in women with polycystic ovary syndrome (PCOS). Fertil Steril. 2010 Jun;94(1):357-9.

[29] Deeks AA, Gibson-Helm ME, Paul E, Teede HJ. Is having polycystic ovary syndrome a predictor of poor psychological function including anxiety and depression? Hum Reprod. 2011 Jun;26(6):1399-407.

[30] Deeks AA, Gibson-Helm ME, Teede HJ. Anxiety and depression in polycystic ovary syndrome: a comprehensive investigation. Fertil Steril. 2010 May 1;93(7):2421-3.

[31] Laggari V, Diareme S, Christogiorgos S, Deligeoroglou E, Christopoulos P, Tsiantis J, et al. Anxiety and depression in adolescents with polycystic ovary syndrome and Mayer-Rokitansky-Kuster-Hauser syndrome. J Psychosom Obstet Gynaecol. 2009 Jun;30(2):83-8.

[32] Hollinrake E, Abreu A, Maifeld M, Van Voorhis BJ, Dokras A. Increased risk of depressive disorders in women with polycystic ovary syndrome. Fertil Steril. 2007 Jun;87(6):1369-76.

[33] Rasgon NL, Rao RC, Hwang S, Altshuler LL, Elman S, Zuckerbrow-Miller J, et al. Depression in women with polycystic ovary syndrome: clinical and biochemical correlates. J Affect Disord. 2003 May;74(3):299-304.

[34] Petersen RW, Quinlivan JA. Preventing anxiety and depression in gynaecological cancer: a randomised controlled trial. Bjog. 2002 Apr;109(4):386-94.

[35] Weiner CL, Primeau M, Ehrmann DA. Androgens and mood dysfunction in women: comparison of women with polycystic ovarian syndrome to healthy controls. Psychosom Med. 2004 May-Jun;66(3):356-62.

[36] Livadas S, Chaskou S, Kandaraki AA, Skourletos G, Economou F, Christou M, et al. Anxiety is associated with hormonal and metabolic profile in women with polycystic ovarian syndrome. Clin Endocrinol (Oxf). 2011 May 23.

[37] Farrell K, Antoni MH. Insulin resistance, obesity, inflammation, and depression in polycystic ovary syndrome: biobehavioral mechanisms and interventions. Fertil Steril. 2010 Oct;94(5):1565-74.

[38] Rofey DL, Szigethy EM, Noll RB, Dahl RE, Lobst E, Arslanian SA. Cognitive-behavioral therapy for physical and emotional disturbances in adolescents with polycystic ovary syndrome: a pilot study. J Pediatr Psychol. 2009 Mar;34(2):156-63.

[39] Vgontzas AN, Legro RS, Bixler EO, Grayev A, Kales A, Chrousos GP. Polycystic ovary syndrome is associated with obstructive sleep apnea and daytime sleepiness: role of insulin resistance. J Clin Endocrinol Metab. 2001 Feb;86(2):517-20.

[40] de Niet JE, de Koning CM, Pastoor H, Duivenvoorden HJ, Valkenburg O, Ramakers MJ, et al. Psychological well-being and sexarche in women with polycystic ovary syndrome. Hum Reprod. 2010 Jun;25(6):1497-503.

[41] Sonino N, Fava GA, Mani E, Belluardo P, Boscaro M. Quality of life of hirsute women. Postgrad Med J. 1993 Mar;69(809):186-9.

[42] Jedel E, Gustafson D, Waern M, Sverrisdottir YB, Landen M, Janson PO, et al. Sex steroids, insulin sensitivity and sympathetic nerve activity in relation to affective symptoms in women with polycystic ovary syndrome. Psychoneuroendocrinology. 2011 May 5.

[43] Kerchner A, Lester W, Stuart SP, Dokras A. Risk of depression and other mental health disorders in women with polycystic ovary syndrome: a longitudinal study. Fertil Steril. 2009 Jan;91(1):207-12.

[44] Barry JA, Hardiman PJ, Saxby BK, Kuczmierczyk A. Testosterone and mood dysfunction in women with polycystic ovarian syndrome compared to subfertile controls. J Psychosom Obstet Gynaecol. 2011 Jun;32(2):104-11.

[45] Benson S, Arck PC, Tan S, Hahn S, Mann K, Rifaie N, et al. Disturbed stress responses in women with polycystic ovary syndrome. Psychoneuroendocrinology. 2009 Jun;34(5):727-35.

[46] Lawrance K, Byers E. Sexual satisfaction in long term heterosexual relationships: the interpersonal exchange model of sexual satisfaction. . Personal Relationships. 1995;2(4):267-85. .

[47] Rosen R, Brown C, Heiman J, Leiblum S, Meston C, Shabsigh R, et al. The Female Sexual Function Index (FSFI): a multidimensional self-report instrument for the assessment of female sexual function. J Sex Marital Ther. 2000 Apr-Jun;26(2):191-208.

[48] Bancroft J, Sanders D, Davidson D, Warner P. Mood, sexuality, hormones, and the menstrual cycle. III. Sexuality and the role of androgens. Psychosom Med. 1983 Dec;45(6):509-16.

[49] Leiblum SR, Rosen RC. Introduction: changing perspectives on sexual desire. Leiblum SR, Rosen RC (ed), Sexual Desire Disorders: New York: Guilford Press 1988.

[50] Toledano R, Pfaus J. The Sexual Arousal and Desire Inventory (SADI): a multidimensional scale to assess subjective sexual arousal and desire. The journal of sexual medicine. 2006 Sep;3(5):853-77.

[51] Laan E, van Driel EM, van Lunsen RH. Genital responsiveness in healthy women with and without sexual arousal disorder. The journal of sexual medicine. 2008 Jun;5(6):1424-35.

[52] Laan E, van Lunsen RH. Hormones and sexuality in postmenopausal women: a psychophysiological study. J Psychosom Obstet Gynaecol. 1997 Jun;18(2):126-33.

[53] Wierman ME, Nappi RE, Avis N, Davis SR, Labrie F, Rosner W, et al. Endocrine aspects of women's sexual function. The journal of sexual medicine. 2010 Jan;7(1 Pt 2):561-85.

[54] Wylie K, Rees M, Hackett G, Anderson R, Bouloux PM, Cust M, et al. Androgens, health and sexuality in women and men. Human fertility (Cambridge, England). 2010 Dec;13(4):277-97.

[55] World Health Organisation. WHO manual for the standardized investigation and diagnosis of the infertile couple. Cambridge: Cambridge University Press 1993.

[56] van Lunsen R. Libido bestaat niet en seks werkt anders dan u denkt! Slager, E (red) Reproductieve geneeskunde, gynaeocologie en obstretie anno 2009. 2009 465-72.

[57] Basson R. A model of women's sexual arousal. J Sex Marital Ther. 2002 Jan-Feb;28(1):1-10.

[58] Basson R, Brotto LA, Petkau AJ, Labrie F. Role of androgens in women's sexual dysfunction. Menopause (New York, NY. 2010 Sep-Oct;17(5):962-71.

[59] Stuckey BG. Female sexual function and dysfunction in the reproductive years: the influence of endogenous and exogenous sex hormones. The journal of sexual medicine. 2008 Oct;5(10):2282-90.
[60] Caruso S, Rugolo S, Agnello C, Romano M, Cianci A. Quality of sexual life in hyperandrogenic women treated with an oral contraceptive containing chlormadinone acetate. The journal of sexual medicine. 2009 Dec;6(12):3376-84.
[61] Bancroft J. Sexual effects of androgens in women: some theoretical considerations. Fertil Steril. 2002 Apr;77 Suppl 4:S55-9.
[62] Basson R. Women's sexual dysfunction: revised and expanded definitions. Cmaj. 2005 May 10;172(10):1327-33.
[63] Basson R. Women's sexual function and dysfunction: current uncertainties, future directions. International journal of impotence research. 2008 Sep-Oct;20(5):466-78.
[64] Both S, Spiering M, Everaerd W, Laan E. Sexual behavior and responsiveness to sexual stimuli following laboratory-induced sexual arousal. Journal of sex research. 2004 Aug;41(3):242-58.
[65] Hahn S, Benson S, Elsenbruch S, Pleger K, Tan S, Mann K, et al. Metformin treatment of polycystic ovary syndrome improves health-related quality-of-life, emotional distress and sexuality. Hum Reprod. 2006 Jul;21(7):1925-34.
[66] Mansson M, Norstrom K, Holte J, Landin-Wilhelmsen K, Dahlgren E, Landen M. Sexuality and psychological wellbeing in women with polycystic ovary syndrome compared with healthy controls. European journal of obstetrics, gynecology, and reproductive biology. 2011 Apr;155(2):161-5.
[67] Pagidas K, Carson SA, McGovern PG, Barnhart HX, Myers ER, Legro RS, et al. Body mass index and intercourse compliance. Fertil Steril. 2010 Sep;94(4):1447-50.
[68] Conaglen HM, Conaglen JV. Sexual desire in women presenting for antiandrogen therapy. J Sex Marital Ther. 2003 Jul-Aug;29(4):255-67.
[69] Gorzynski G, Katz JL. The polycystic ovary syndrome:psychosexual correlates. Arch Sex Behav. 1977 May;6(3):215-22.
[70] Battaglia C, Nappi RE, Mancini F, Cianciosi A, Persico N, Busacchi P, et al. PCOS, sexuality, and clitoral vascularisation: a pilot study. The journal of sexual medicine. 2008 Dec;5(12):2886-94.
[71] Davis SR, Davison SL, Donath S, Bell RJ. Circulating androgen levels and self-reported sexual function in women. Jama. 2005 Jul 6;294(1):91-6.
[72] Kadioglu P, Yetkin DO, Sanli O, Yalin AS, Onem K, Kadioglu A. Obesity might not be a risk factor for female sexual dysfunction. BJU international. 2010 Nov;106(9):1357-61.
[73] Manlove HA, Guillermo C, Gray PB. Do women with polycystic ovary syndrome (PCOS) report differences in sex-typed behavior as children and adolescents?: Results of a pilot study. Annals of human biology. 2008 Nov-Dec;35(6):584-95.
[74] Smith HA, Markovic N, Matthews AK, Danielson ME, Kalro BN, Youk AO, et al. A comparison of polycystic ovary syndrome and related factors between lesbian and heterosexual women. Womens Health Issues. 2011 May-Jun;21(3):191-8.
[75] Agrawal R, Sharma S, Bekir J, Conway G, Bailey J, Balen AH, et al. Prevalence of polycystic ovaries and polycystic ovary syndrome in lesbian women compared with heterosexual women. Fertil Steril. 2004 Nov;82(5):1352-7.

[76] Bosinski HA, Peter M, Bonatz G, Arndt R, Heidenreich M, Sippell WG, et al. A higher rate of hyperandrogenic disorders in female-to-male transsexuals. Psychoneuroendocrinology. 1997 Jul; 22(5):361-80.
[77] Rotterdam EA-SPCWG. Revised 2003 consensus on diagnostic criteria and long-term health risks related to polycystic ovary syndrome. Fertil Steril. 2004 Jan;81(1):19-25.
[78] Ferriman D, Gallwey JD. Clinical assessment of body hair growth in women. J Clin Endocrinol Metab. 1961 Nov;21:1440-7.
[79] Schmitt DP, Allik J. Simultaneous administration of the Rosenberg Self-Esteem Scale in 53 nations: exploring the universal and culture-specific features of global self-esteem. J Pers Soc Psychol. 2005 Oct;89(4):623-42.
[80] Secord PF, Jourard SM. The appraisal of body-cathexis: body-cathexis and the self. J Consult Psychol. 1953 Oct;17(5):343-7.
[81] Baardman I, de Jong JG. Measuring Body Cathexis. Bewegen & Hulpverlening. 1984;1:28–41.
[82] Leary MR. A brief version of the Fear of Negative Evaluation Scale. Personality and Social Psychology Bulletin. 1983;9 371–5.
[83] Graaf de H, Meijer S, Poelman J, Vanwesenbeeck I. Seksuele gezondheid van jongeren in Nederland anno 2005. Uitgeverij Eburon, Delft. 2005.
[84] Sterne JA, White IR, Carlin JB, Spratt M, Royston P, Kenward MG, et al. Multiple imputation for missing data in epidemiological and clinical research: potential and pitfalls. Bmj. 2009;338:b2393.
[85] Dempster A, Laird N, Rubin D. Maximum likelihood from incomplete data via the EM algorithm. . Journal of the Royal Statistical Society, Series B. 1997(39):174-94.
[86] Conaglen JV, Conaglen HM. The effects of treating male hypogonadism on couples' sexual desire and function. The journal of sexual medicine. 2009 Feb;6(2):456-63.
[87] Collins RL, Kashdan TB, Gollnisch G. The feasibility of using cellular phones to collect ecological momentary assessment data: application to alcohol consumption. Experimental and clinical psychopharmacology. 2003 Feb;11(1):73-8.
[88] Kvalem IL, von Soest T, Traeen B, Singsaas K. Body evaluation and coital onset: a population-based longitudinal study. Body image. 2011 Mar;8(2):110-8.
[89] Burri A, Spector T. Recent and Lifelong Sexual Dysfunction in a Female UK Population Sample: Prevalence and Risk Factors. The journal of sexual medicine. 2011 Jun 15.
[90] Dokras A, Clifton S, Futterweit W, Wild R. Increased risk for abnormal depression scores in women with polycystic ovary syndrome: a systematic review and meta-analysis. Obstetrics and gynecology. 2011 Jan;117(1):145-52.
[91] Skrzypulec V, Drosdzol A. Evaluation of the quality of life and sexual functioning of women using a 30-microg ethinyloestradiol and 3-mg drospirenone combined oral contraceptive. Eur J Contracept Reprod Health Care. 2008 Mar;13(1):49-57.
[92] Hoeger K. Obesity and weight loss in polycystic ovary syndrome. Obstet Gynecol Clin North Am. 2001 Mar;28(1):85-97, vi-vii.
[93] Norman RJ, Homan G, Moran L, Noakes M. Lifestyle choices, diet, and insulin sensitizers in polycystic ovary syndrome. Endocrine. 2006 Aug;30(1):35-43.
[94] Andersen P, Seljeflot I, Abdelnoor M, Arnesen H, Dale PO, Lovik A, et al. Increased insulin sensitivity and fibrinolytic capacity after dietary intervention in obese women with polycystic ovary syndrome. Metabolism. 1995 May;44(5):611-6.

[95] Clark AM, Thornley B, Tomlinson L, Galletley C, Norman RJ. Weight loss in obese infertile women results in improvement in reproductive outcome for all forms of fertility treatment. Hum Reprod. 1998 Jun;13(6):1502-5.
[96] Kiddy DS, Hamilton-Fairley D, Bush A, Short F, Anyaoku V, Reed MJ, et al. Improvement in endocrine and ovarian function during dietary treatment of obese women with polycystic ovary syndrome. Clin Endocrinol (Oxf). 1992 Jan;36(1):105-11.
[97] Galletly C, Moran L, Noakes M, Clifton P, Tomlinson L, Norman R. Psychological benefits of a high-protein, low-carbohydrate diet in obese women with polycystic ovary syndrome--a pilot study. Appetite. 2007 Nov;49(3):590-3.
[98] Keegan A, Liao LM, Boyle M. 'Hirsutism': a psychological analysis. J Health Psychol. 2003 May;8(3):327-45.
[99] Clayton WJ, Lipton M, Elford J, Rustin M, Sherr L. A randomized controlled trial of laser treatment among hirsute women with polycystic ovary syndrome. Br J Dermatol. 2005 May;152(5):986-92.
[100] Percy CA, Gibbs T, Potter L, Boardman S. Nurse-led peer support group: experiences of women with polycystic ovary syndrome. J Adv Nurs. 2009 Oct;65(10):2046-55.
[101] Bitzer J, Platano G, Tschudin S, Alder J. Sexual counseling for women in the context of physical diseases: a teaching model for physicians. The journal of sexual medicine. 2007 Jan;4(1):29-37.
[102] Annon J. Behavioral treatment of sexual problems. Harper & Row. 1976.

3

Android Subcutaneous Adipose Tissue Topography in Females with Polycystic Ovary Syndrome: A Visible Phenotype Even in Juveniles

Moeller Reinhard, Giuliani Albrecht, Mangge Harald, Tafeit Erwin, Glaeser Margit, Schrabmair Walter and Horejsi Renate
Medical University Graz
Austria

1. Introduction

Polycystic Ovary-Syndrome (PCOS) is a complex endocrine disorder which affects approximately 5-10% of females of reproductive age (Asunción et al, 2000, Diamanti-Kandarakis et al, 1999, Dunaif A, 1997). The syndrome is characterized by abnormal menstrual cyclicity, ovulatory dysfunction, hyperandrogenism and hirsutism (Goodarzi et al, 2011, Hatch et al, 1981). Functional ovarian hyperandrogenism is due to hyperinsulinemia, insulin resistance and hyperlipidemia. The acute problems of the patient, namely ovarian abnormalities and ovulation induction for subfertility, have shifted toward the prevention of long-term health consequences (Cupisti et al, 2007). Insulin resistance is a key feature of females with PCOS, especially, when they are overweight or obese. This has important effects in favouring androgen excess and oligo-anovulation. It is evident, that females with PCOS, especially the overweight ones, have a higher risk for developing type 2 diabetes. It is suggested, that insulin resistance is even more common in overweight patients with PCOS that in lean females. There is a continuum of decrease in insulin sensitivity with increasing abdominal fat accumulation (Zelzer et al, 2011). Hyperandrogenism is associated with fat accumulation at the body trunk. This android, "apple"-like fat pattern is a risk for metabolic disturbances like cardiovascular diseases and type 2 diabetes (Cupisti et al, 2007, Nathan & Moran, 2008).

Early symptoms of PCOS such as growing precociously pubic hair, height growth and overweight, do already appear during childhood and adolescence, but the problems are not diagnosed seriously (Bronstein et al, 2011, Oliveira et al, 2010). Obesity in childhood is widely spread worldwide. Lower physical activity and a general availability of high caloric food may cause high proportions of overweight and obese juveniles for higher risks for females to develop PCOS.

Females with PCOS need medical care for different reasons: the pediatrician may be contacted because of childhood obesity or abnormal menstrual bleeding. The dermatologist may be approached for hirsutism. The gynecologist may be consulted for menstrual cycle abnormalities, unfulfilled wish for pregnancy, or complications during pregnancy. The physician of internal medicine may be consulted for obesity or type 2 diabetes. The cause of a first contact of the patient with a physician is often a rapid weight gain. The consulted physician will measure BMI or waist circumference. The suggestion of metabolic terms, however, should focus the interest on the distribution of body fat, not only on body weight. A rapid, non-invasive and precise measurement of the thickness of adipose tissue might render important information of metabolic risks even in juveniles and in young females. Advanced statistic methods could support the detection of a PCOS - like fat distribution and confirm the risk for metabolic disturbances (Tafeit et al, 2000; Tafeit et al, 2000a, Tafeit et al, 1999).

2. The lipometer

Measuring body fat has increasing priority in medical care, but also in sports and human biology. The standard methods are caliper, computed tomography, underwater weighing, nuclear magnetic resonance, bio-impedance or dual energy X-ray absoptiometry (DEXA). These methods have several disadvantages like high costs, stress for the subject, radiological burden or lack of precision.

The newly certificated optical device Lipometer is a computerized optical system for precise measurement of the absolute thicknesses of subcutaneous adipose tissue in mm (Tafeit et al, 2000b).

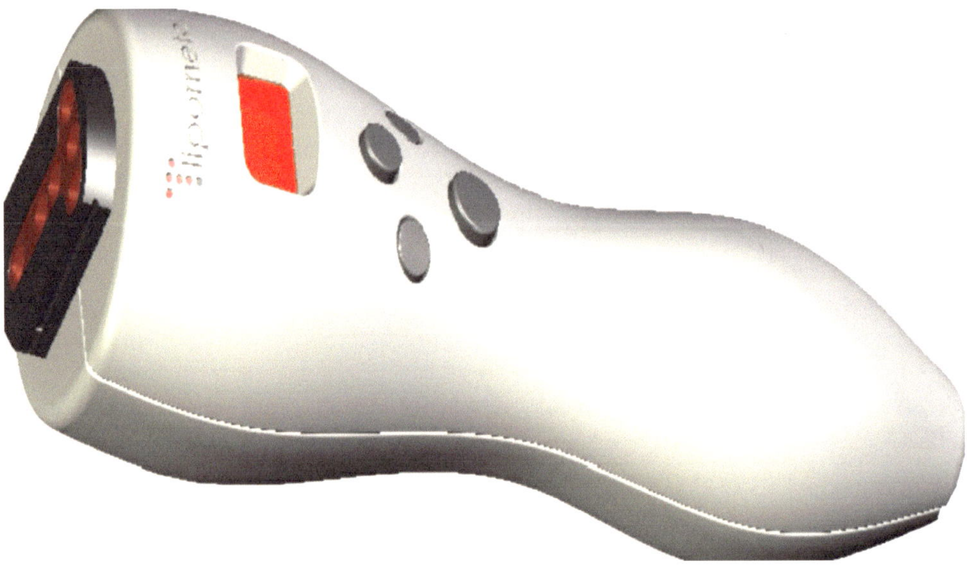

Fig. 1. The Lipometer, an optical device to measure the thickness of subcutaneous adipose tissue layers

2.1 Design of the lipometer

The sensor head of the Lipometer consists of five light-emitting diodes as light sources (wavelength 660 nm, light intensity 3000 mcd) and a photodetector. The diodes illuminate the body site to be measured, forming geometrical patterns that vary in succession. The light intensities from the adipose tissue are back-scattered, amplified, digitized and render fat thickness of the named body site in mm (Moeller at al, 2000). Calibration and evaluation was done by computed tomography as reference method.

2.2 Procedere of measuring Subcutaneous Adipose Tissue Topography (SAT-Top)

Fifteen anatomically well defined body sites from 1-neck to 15-calf give the information of individual body fat distribution (Subcutaneous adipose tissue topography, SAT-Top) (Tafeit et al, 2007). The coefficient of variation of these 15 body sites was published previously (Sudi et al, 2000).

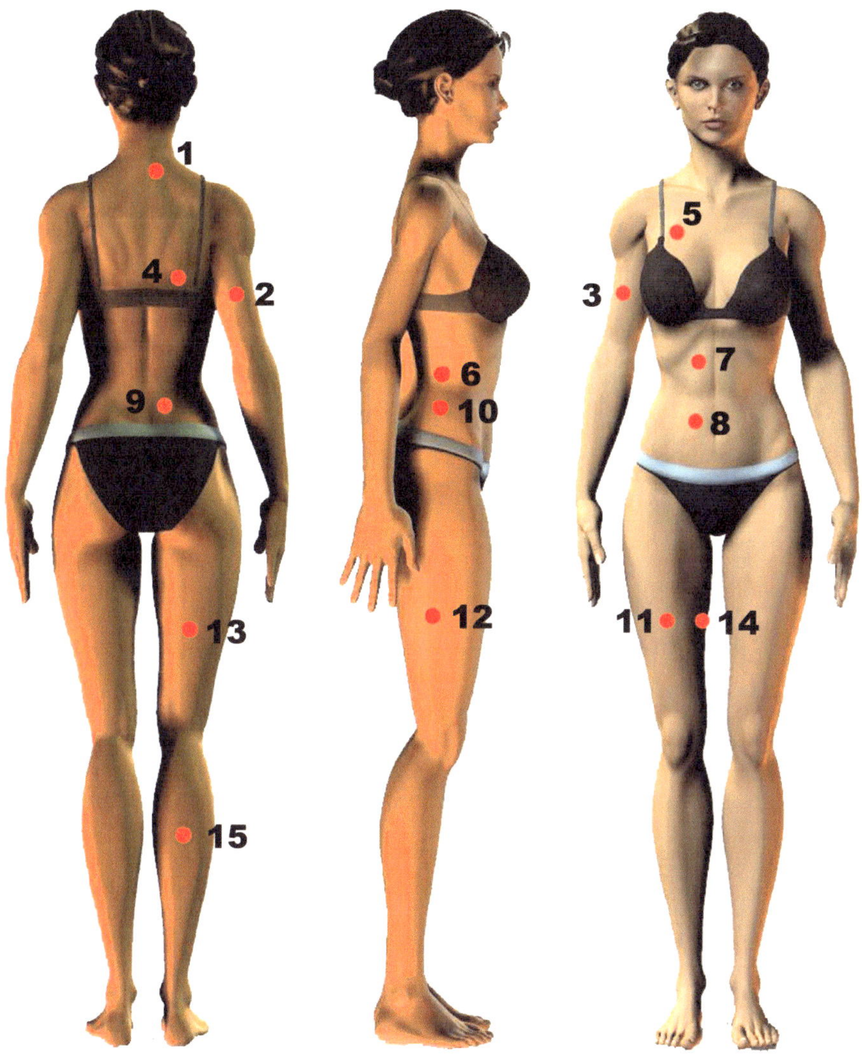

Fig. 2. The set of fifteen anatomically well- defined body sites from 1-neck to 15-calf on the right side oft the human body

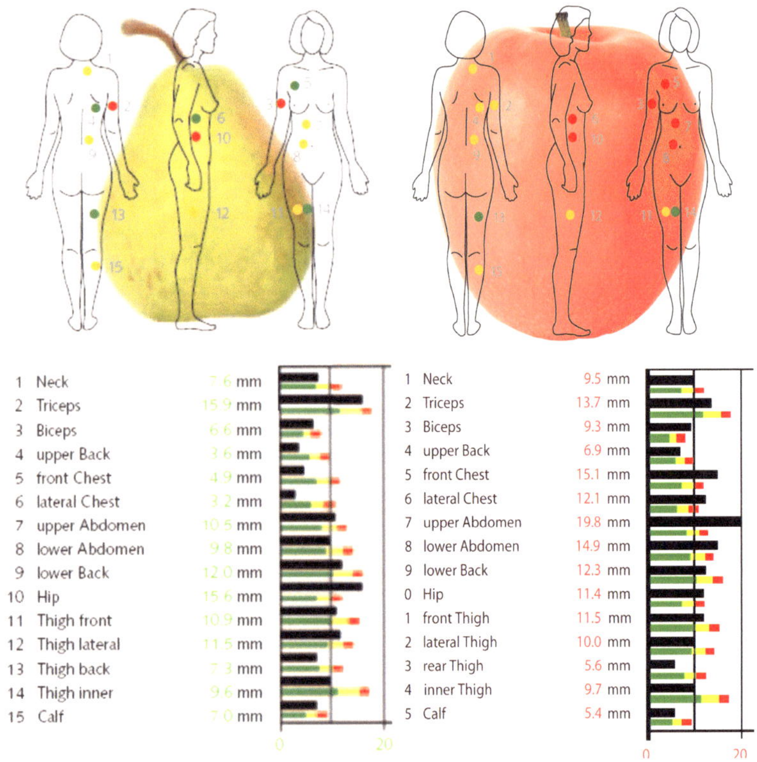

Fig. 3. SAT-Top protocols: Female pear profile (left) and female apple profile (right) with the same age, weight and BMI

SAT-Top of the measured person is like an individual "fingerprint", defined by genetics, sex, nutritional status, hormonal and metabolic disorders and modified by age and life style.

2.3 Comparing an individually measured SAT-Top with the data of healthy or diseased subjects of the same sex and age

SAT-Tops of more than 3000 men, women and children are included in the Lipometer data base, healthy subjects as well as patients with type 2 diabetes, coronary heart disease, obesity and fertility disorders (Moeller et al, 2000a).

Both, male and female children develop about the same SAT-Top between birth and the age before the onset of puberty. At the age of about eleven years the adipose tissue layers on the extremities increase in girls. The maximum of the adipose tissue layers on the legs is reached at the age of 22 years. Boys, however, decrease the thicknesses of the subcutaneous adipose tissue layers at the extremities. The minimum of the thickness of adipose tissue layers at the extremities is reached at the age of 17 years.

At the age of 20 years men and women increase adipose tissue layers at their trunks until they are about 60 years old. Men have skinny extremities, women have not.

In later life man and women stop increasing the thicknesses of adipose tissue layers at the trunks and turn back to thinner layers at their trunks.

Patients with obesity, type 2 diabetes, coronary heart disease, PCOS and anorexia nervosa have significantly different SAT-Tops compared to age-matched healthy controls. Anorectic patients have not the typical patterns of a male or female body fat distribution, but all over the body extremely thin adipose tissue layers of somewhat less than one mm. Overweight patients increase adipose tissue layers on neck, trunk, abdomen, hip and back and accumulate visceral fat, the "apple"-like body fat distribution. An even more pronounced "super- apple"- like body silhouette can also be found in overweight PCOS women and patients with type 2 diabetes and coronary heart disease (Moeller et al, 2000).

3. Polycystic Ovary Syndrome and body fat distribution

The diagnosis of PCOS is based on the Rotterdam criteria (The Rotterdam ESHRE-ASRM-Sponsored consensus workshop group, 2004). Two out of three of the following are required for the diagnosis: oligo- and/or anovulation, clinical and/or biochemical signs of hyperandrogenism, polycystic ovaries by ultrasound. Disorders with a similar clinical presentation have to be excluded.

About half of the females with PCOS are overweight or obese. The body fat distribution and SAT-Top is a better indicator of metabolic changes than waist circumference or BMI. Hyperandrogenism can be attributed to a fat accumulation at the trunk (Enea et al, 2011). Females with an android body silhouette have a higher risk for developing cardiovascular diseases, or type 2 diabetes (Goodarzi et al, 2011).

3.1 SAT-Top comparison of adult females

SAT-Top was measured in healthy females, overweight and lean females with PCOS. Diagnosis was performed by the Division of Reproductive Endocrinology of the Medical University Graz because of unfulfilled wish of pregnancy. Polycystic ovaries were diagnosed by ultrasound. Oligo- and anovulation, acne or alopecia and /or elevated androgen levels were identified (Hatch et al, 1981).

	healthy controls	obese PCOS	lean PCOS
N	87	18	15
Age (years)	28,1±4,1	27,3±4,9	25,6±4,1
Height (cm)	165,5±6,6	164,5±6,5	165,8±8,3
Weight (kg)	60±9,4	83,9±13,6	56,8±7,6
BMI (kg/m^2)	21,9±2,9	31,0±4,7	20,7±2,3

Table 1. Personal data of adult females

The green area in figure 4 shows the body fat distribution of healthy females, a typical "pear"-like body fat distribution with thicker adipose tissue layers at the extremities: triceps and legs.

Lean young females with PCOS (orange bars in figure 4) have thinner adipose tissue layers over the whole body and relatively thin layers at the extremities, but the profile is still more "pear"-like.

Overweight and obese females with PCOS (red bars in the figure) have a remarkable different body fat distribution with significantly thicker fat layers at all body sites from neck to hip and thinner layers at their legs, a typical "apple"- like body fat distribution (Tafeit et al, 2003).

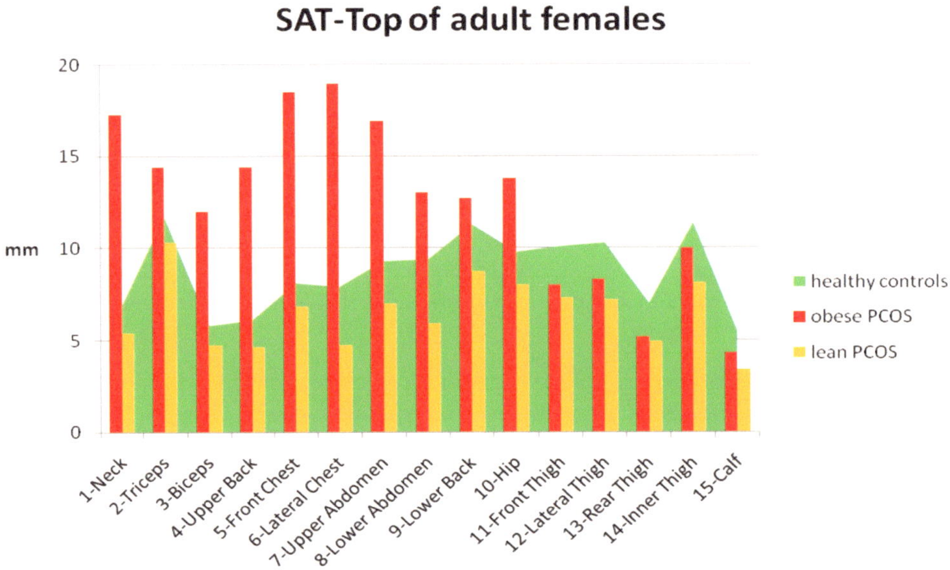

Fig. 4. SAT-Tops of healthy control females (green area), obese women with PCOS (red bars) and lean women with PCOS (orange bars)

3.2 Body fat distribution of women with type 2 diabetes

SAT-Top of 20 women with type 2 diabetes was published previously and the subcutaneous body fat pattern has strong similarities to obese women with PCOS.

The personal data are shown in table 2:

	healthy women	type 2 diabetes
N	122	20
Age (years)	58,1±6,2	62,4±6,6
Height (cm)	161,9±5,9	160,9±5,4
Weight (kg)	72,1±11,6	75,4±13,1
BMI (kg/m^2)	27,5±4,5	29,1±4,9

Table 2. Personal data of elderly females

Figure 5 shows SAT-Tops of healthy controls (green area) compared to those with type 2 diabetes (violet bars):

The healthy elderly controls have increased thicknesses of adipose tissue layers located at the trunk during the postmenopausal aging processes. Overthere females with type 2 diabetes develop thicker fat layers at their trunks, while the extremities are thinner than that of healthy elderly controls (Tafeit et al, 2000).

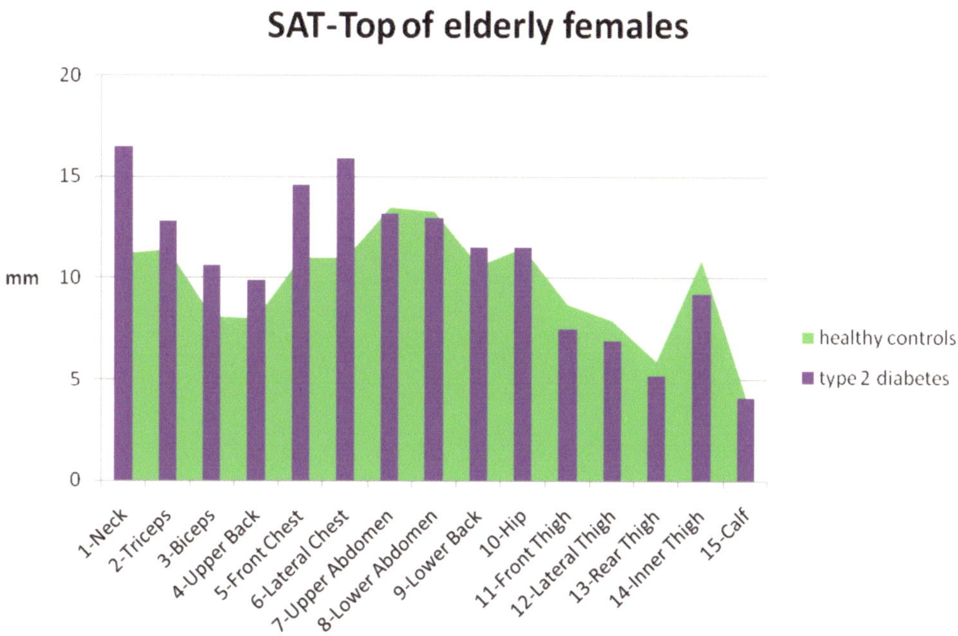

Fig. 5. SAT-Tops of healthy elderly controls (green area) and elderly females with type 2 diabetes (violet bars).

3.3 Body fat distribution of normal weight and overweight young girls

SAT-Top was measured in 25 overweight, female juveniles and age-matched controls.

The table shows the personal data:

	healthy controls	overweight girls
N	301	25
Age (years)	12,6±1,3	13,1±0,3
Height (cm)	156±9,2	160±6,1
Weight (kg)	46,8±10,8	78,8±12,3
BMI (kg/m^2)	19,3±3,0	30,8±4,7

Table 3. Personal data of adolescent females

Figure 6 shows the SAT-profiles of healthy (green area) and overweight (pink bars) female juveniles at the age of 13 years:

Healthy girls begin to develop a gynoid body silhouette with thicker fat layers at the extremities. The overweight girls have thicker adipose tissue layers at all measured body sites, including also at the extremities. The body sites at the trunk are significantly thicker than those of the healthy controls. The body fat distribution of those juveniles is comparable to 60-years–old females with type 2 diabetes and adult females with PCOS (Tafeit et al, 2000, Moeller et al, 2007).

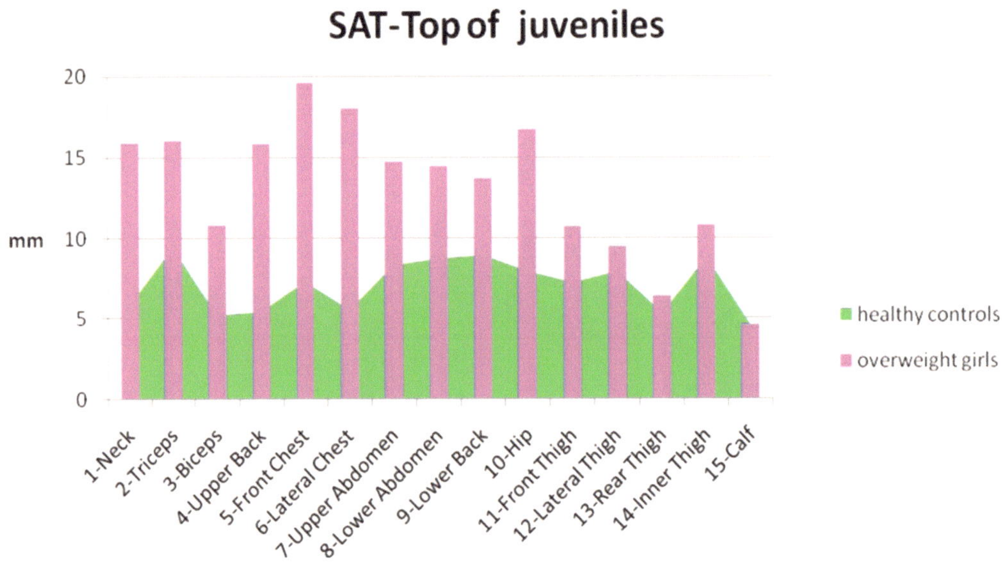

Fig. 6. SAT-Tops of healthy young girls (green area) and overweight girls (pink bars)

3.4 Comparison of the three groups of patients

The presented groups of patients (obese young females with PCOS, elderly females with type 2 diabetes and obese young girls) have an "apple"-like body fat distribution. Insulin resistance is suggested and consistently high risk for meatabolic diseases. The comparison of their SAT-Top plots is shown in figure 7:

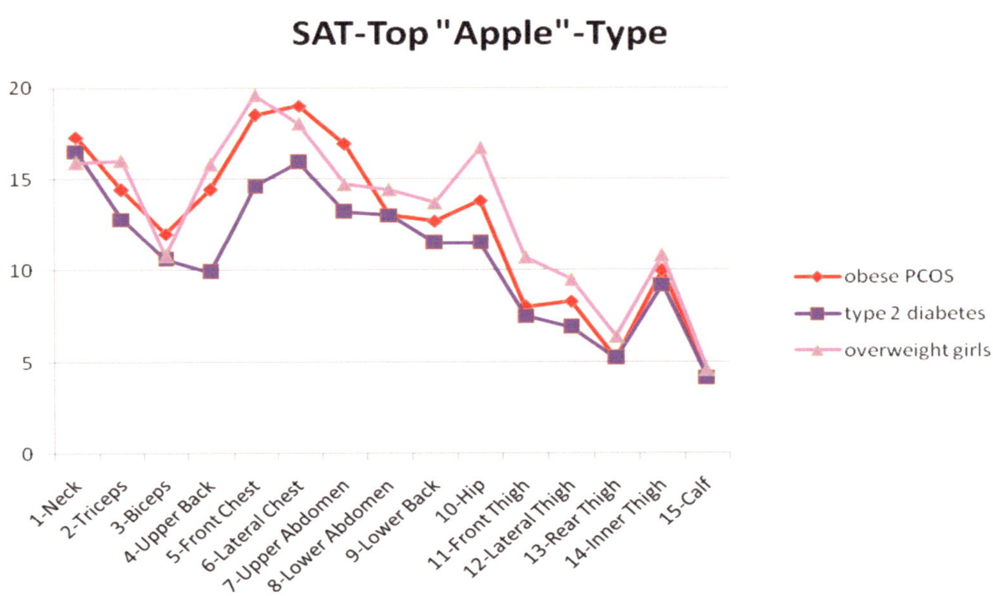

Fig. 7. SAT-Tops of obese females with PCOS (red line), females with type 2 diabetes (violet line) and overweight girls (pink line)

The "apple"- like body fat distribution is nearly congruent in females at the age of 13 years (overweight girls), 27 years (females with PCOS) and 62 years (females with type 2 diabetes).

Factor analysis condenses the 15-dimensional information of SAT-Top data in a two-dimensional diagram. Factor 1, the x-axis, represents the combined measured data of the trunk, Factor 2, the y-axis, represents the data of the extremities. The blue line in the figure is the development healthy male controls from 9 (m09) to 80 years (m80). A 9 years old boy has thin fat layers at the trunk. To the age of 17 years the young male decreases the thickness of adipose tissue layers at the extremities. Between the age of 17 years to 40 years the young male increases fat layers on the trunk (m17, m22, m30, m40). Between 40 and 60 years male individuals turn back to thinner trunk layers (m40, m50, m60).

The red line shows the development of SAT-Top in females from 9 (f09) to 80 (f80) years. A 9 years-old girl has lean extremities and thin fat layers at the trunk. The thickness of adipose tissue layers at the extremities increases till the age of 22 (f22). Between 22 years and 60 years female persons increase their fat layers at their trunks and decrease it in older age between 60 and 80 years (f60 –f80).

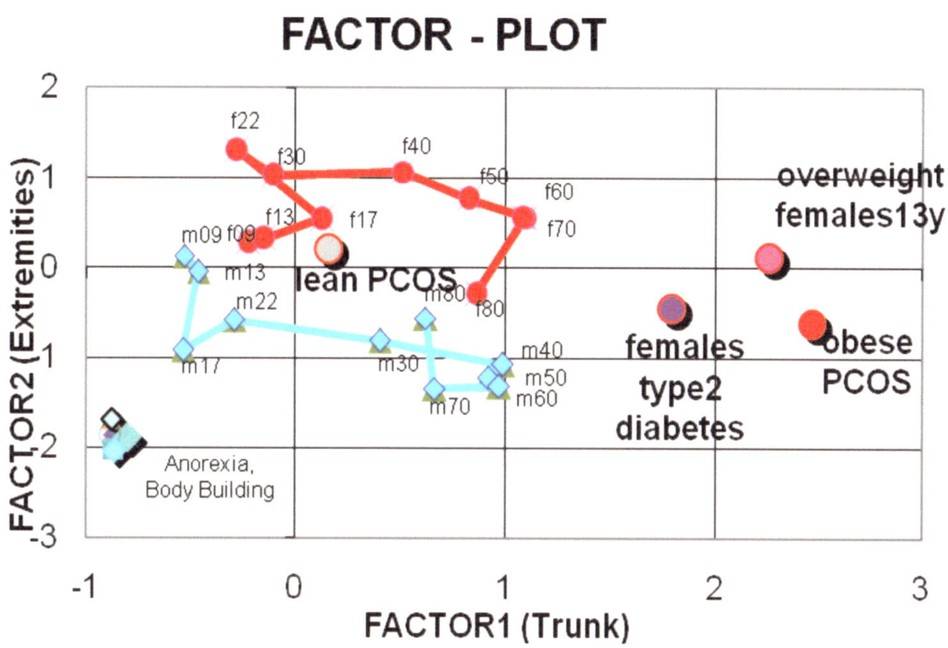

Fig. 8. Factor analysis condenses the SAT-Top information at the trunk and the body sites at the extremities into a two-dimensional plot, where the position of each subject can be shown.

The gynoid body silhouette seen in fertile young females is a signal reproductive potential. Regarding SAT-Top of females with PCOS, a high divergence of the typical femal body silhouette is evident.

All SAT-Top plots shown in this chapter indicate, that almost all SAT layers of the upper body were significantly thicker in obese adolescents, obese females with PCOS and elderly females with type 2 diabetes, whereas SAT-layers at the legs were thinner compared to healthy controls of the same age group.

The patients described in this chapter, namely overweight females with PCOS, females with type 2 diabetes and overweight female adolescents are positioned at higher values of Factor 1, indicating significantly thicker adipose tissue layers at the trunk. Factor 2, the condensed body sites at the extremities show lower values in females with PCOS and type 2 diabetes compared to the age matched control group.

4. Conclusion

PCOS is a common disorder, representing an early indication of future metabolic risks (Barber & Franks, 2010, Sloboda et al, 2011). Obese females with PCOS have more severe clinical features than normal weight females with PCOS (lean PCOS) (Pandey & Bhattacharya, 2010). Because of the world-wide epidemic increase of obesity the prevalence of PCOS appears to be rising, too. Overweight and obesity have a profound effect on the clinical manifestation of insulin resistance, PCOS, and type 2 diabetes. Females and adolescents with PCOS suffer also from psychicals burdens such as feeling less attractive than peers, they have less sexual contacts also because of obesity and hirsutism.

Insulin resistance is a condition of PCOS. Insulin resistance promotes fat storage because glucose is not taken by the cells. Increased levels of insulin in the blood stream cause wide-ranging consequences that can lead to a variety of other serious health conditions, such as coronary heart disease, hypertension, diabetes, as well as infertility, abnormal hair growth, cysts on the ovaries. These high insulin levels in the blood even in young girls are correlated to abdominal fat accumulation, which is highly difficult to demolish. Recent studies confirm that caloric intake and energy expenditure is at a comparable range in healthy and insulin resistant subjects. Therefore loosing weight and decreasing abdominal fat is a long-term and often frustrating process. Otherwise - it is highly important for females with PCOS and overweight adolescent girls to induce weight loss and fat loss in the abdominal area; more than in the general population (Hrzystek-Korpacka et al, 2011). Body weight loss is associated with beneficial effects on the clinical features. Insulin-sensitizing agents might support weight reduction programs (Grover & Yialamas, 2011). The named patients (juvenile females, overweight young women with PCOS and elderly women with type 2 diabetes) should receive any support for weight loss (fat loss) by their practitioner. Especially the early intervention combating obesity in juveniles regarding growth and development stages must become the challenge of health services. Lifestyle modification is a key factor for enhancing quality of life for overweight and anovulatory females. Prior to ovulation induction treatments weight loss should be encouraged. The lower life quality is more attributed to obesity and hirsutism than to psychosocial status and social adjustment (Swallen et al, 2005). Any interventions in PCOS women that reduce trunk fat also influences hirsutism, acne, infertility and overall psychological and emotional condition (Elsenbruch et al, 2003). An individually adapted diet and physical activity should be the first steps in intervention strategies for overweight juveniles and women with PCOS. Early lifestyle interventions cause significantly reduced body fat and androgen levels, and improved insulin sensitivity and menstrual cycles (Norman et al, 2004).

The process of an effective weight-loss management by diet and exercise can be monitored by SAT-Top measurement. The decrease of the thickness of adipose tissue layers might be a motivation factor for the patient to continue and maintain weight loss intervention programs.

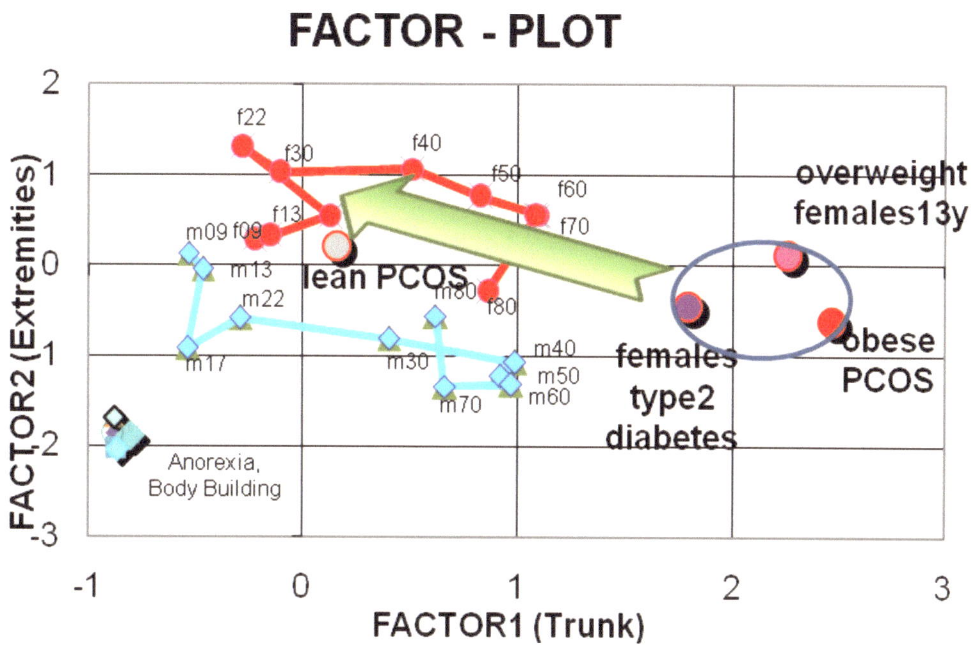

Fig. 9. Expectation of a successfull intervention program: the movement of an" apple"-like SAT-Top to a more "pear"- position in the factor plot (green arrow).

Furthermore, factor analysis of the SAT-Top data can immediately demonstrate, where the position of the patient in the factor plot is located. An effective trunk fat reduction program should move the position of the subject towards the area of healthy controls of the same age.

5. References

Asunción, M., Calvo, R., San Millán, J., Avila, S. & Escobar - Morreale H. (2000). A prospective study of the prevalence of the polycystic ovary syndrome in unselected Caucasian women from Spain. *Journal of Clinical Endocrinology & Metabolism* Vol. 85: pp 2434-2438.

Barber, T .& Franks, S. (2010) Genetic basis of polycystic ovary syndrome. *Expert Review of Endocrinology & Metabolism* Vol 5 (No.4): pp549-561.

Bronstein, J., Tawdekar, S., Liu, Y., Pawelczak, M., David, R. & Shah, B. (2011). Age of onset of polycystic ovarian syndrome in girls may be earlier than previously thought. *Journal of Pediatric & Adolescent Gynecology* Vol. 24 (No.1): pp 15-20.

Cupisti, S., Dittrich, R., Binder, H., Kajaia, N., Hoffmann, I., Maltaris, T. & Beckmann, M. (2007). Influence of body mass index on measured and calculated androgen parameters in adult women with hirsutism and PCOS. *Experimental and Clinical Endocrinology & Diabetes* Vol 115 (No.6): pp 380-386.

Diamanti-Kandarakis, E., Kouli, C., Bergiele, A., Filandra, F., Tsianateli, T. & Spina, G. (1999). A survey oft he polycystic ovary syndrome in the Greek island of Lesbos: hormonal and metabolic profile. *Journal of Clinical Endocrinology & Metabolism.* Vol 84: pp 4006-4011.

Dunaif, A. (1997). Insulin resistance and the polycystic ovary syndrome: mechanisms and implications for pathogenesis. *Endocrine Reviews* . Vol 18: pp 774-800.

Elsenbruch, S., Hahn, S. & Kowalsky, D. (2003) Quality of life, psychosocial well-being, and sexual satisfaction in women with polycystic ovary syndrome. *Journal of Clinical Endocrinlogy & Metabolism.* Vol 88: pp 1551-1557.

Enea, C., Boisseau, N., Fargeas-Gluck, M., Diaz, V. & Dugue B. (2011). Circulating androgens in women: exercise induced changes. *Sports Medicine* Vol 41 (No.1): pp 1-15.

Goodarzi, M., Dumesic, D., Chazenbalk, G. & Azziz, R. (2011). Polycystic Ovary Syndrome: etiology, pathogenesis and diagnosis. *Nature Reviews Endocrinology* Vol 7 (No.4): pp 219-231.

Grover, A. & Yialamas, M.(2011). Reproductive endocrinology: Metformin or thiazolidinedione therapy in PCOS? *Nature Reviews Endocrinology* Vol 7: pp128-129.

Hatch, R., Rosenfield, R., Kim, H.& Tredway D.(1981). Hirsutism: implications, etiology and management. *American Journal of Obstetrics & Gynecology* Vol 114: pp 815-830.

Hrzystek-Korpacka, M., Malgorzata, P., Kustrzeba-Wojcicka, C., Gamian, A & Noczynska A (2011). The effect of a one-year weight reduction program on seruyl uric acid in overweight - obese children and adolescents. *Clinical Chemistry & Laboratory Medicine* Vol 49 : pp 915-921.

Moeller, R., Horejsi, R., Pilz, S., Lang, N., Sargsyan, K., Dimitrova, R., Tafeit, E., Giuliani, A., Almer, G &, Mangge, H.(2007). Evaluation of risk profiles by subcutaneous adipose tissue topography in obese juveniles. *Obesity* Vol 15 (No.5): pp 1319-1324.

Moeller, R., Tafeit, E., Smolle, K., Pieber, T., Ipsiroglu, O., Duesse, M., Huemer, C., Sudi, K. & Reibnegger, G.(2000a). Estimating percentage total body fat and determining subcutaneous adipose tissue distribution with a new noninvasive optical device Lipometer. *American Journal of Human Biology* Vol 12 (No.2) pp 221-230.

Moeller, R.; Tafeit, E.; Sudi, K, & Reibnegger , G. (2000) Quantifying the `appleness´ or `pearness´of the human body by subcutaneous adipose tissue distribution. *Annals of Human Biology* , Vol .27 (No.1): pp 47-55.

Nathan, B. & Moran, A. (2008). Metabolic complications of obesity in childhood and adolescence: more than just diabetes. *Current Opinion in Endocrinology, Diabetes & Obesity* Vol.15 (No.1): pp 21-29.

Norman, R., Noakes, M., Wu, R., Davies, M., Moran, L.& Wang, J. (2004) Improving reproductive performance in overweight/obese women with effective weight management. *Human Reproduction Update* Vol 10: pp 251-257.

Oberfield, S., Sopher, A.& Gerken A.(2011). Approach to the girl with early onset of pubic hair. *Journal of Endcrinology & Metabolism*, Vol 96 (No.6): pp 1610-1622.

Oliveira, A., Sampaio, B., Teixeira, A., Castro-Correia, C., Fontoura, M. & Luis Medina, J. (2010). Polycystic ovary syndrome: challenge in adolescence. *Endocrinologia y Nutricion* Vol 57 (No.7): pp 328-336.

Pandey, S. & Bhattacharya. (2010) Impact of obesity on gynecology. *Women´s Health* Vol 6 (No1): pp 107-117.

Sloboda, D., Hickey, M. & Hart, R.(2011) Reproduction in females: the role of the early life environment. *Human Reproduction Update* Vol 17 (No.2): pp210-227.

Sudi, K., Tafeit, E., Moeller,R., Gallistl, S.& Borkenstein, M.(2000). Relationship between different aubcutaneous adipose tissue layers, fat mass, and leptin in response to short-term energy restriction in obese girls. *American Journal of Human Biology* Vol 12 (No.6): pp 803-813.

Swallen, K., Reither, E., Haas, S. & Meier, A. (2005). Overweight, obesity and health-related quality of life among adolescents: the National Longitudinal Study of Adolescent Health. *Pediatrics*, Vol 115: pp 340-347.

Tafeit, E., Moeller ,R., Sudi, K.& Reibnegger, G.(2000b). Artificial neural networks as a method to improve the precision of subcutaneous adipose tissue thickness measurement s by means oft he optical device Lipometer. *Computers in Biology and Medicine* Vol 30 (No. 6): pp 355-365.

Tafeit, E., Moeller R, Sudi, K., Horejsi, R., Berg, A.& Reibnegger, G.(2001). Orthogonal factor coefficient development of subcutaneous adipose tissue topography (SAT-Top) in girls and boys. *American Journal of Physical Anthropology* Vol 115: pp 57-61.

Tafeit, E., Moeller, R., Giuliani, A., Urdl, W., Freytag, U., Crailsheim, K., Sudi, K &, Horejsi, R. (2003). Subcutaneous adipose tissue pattern in lean and obese women with polycystic ovary syndrome. *Experimental Biology and Medicine* Vol 228: pp 710-716.

Tafeit, E., Moeller, R., Jurimae, T., Sudi, K.& Wallner, S.(2007). Subcutaneous adipose tissue topography (SAT-Top) development in children and young adults. *Collegium Anthropologicum* Vol 31 (No. 2): pp 395-402.

Tafeit, E., Moeller, R., Pieber, T., Sudi, K.& Reibnegger, G. (2000a). Differences of subcutaneous adipose tissue topography in type 2 diabetic women (NIDDM) and healthy controls. *American Journal of Physical Anthropology* Vol 113: pp 381-388.

Tafeit, E., Moeller, R., Sudi, K. & Reibnegger, G. (2000). ROC and CART analysis of subcutaneous adipose tissue topography (SAT-Top) in type 2 diabetic women and healthy females. *American Journal of Human Biology* Vol 12 (No. 3): pp 388-394.

Tafeit, E., Moeller, R., Sudi, K.& Reibnegger, G. (1999). The determination of three subcutaneous adipose tissue compartments in non –insulin dependent diabetes mellitus women with artificial neural networks and factor analysis . *Artificial Intelligence in Medicine* Vol 17 (No. 2): pp 181-193.

The Rotterdam ESHRE-ASRM-Sponsored consensus workshop group. Revised consensous diagnostic criteria and long-term health risk related to polycystic ovary syndrome (PCOS)(2004). *Human Reproduction* Vol 19, pp 41-47.

Zelzer, S., Fuchs, N., Almer, G.,Raggam, R.,Prueller, F., Truschnig-Wilders, M., Schnedl, W. Horejsi, R., Moeller, R.,Weghuber, D., Ille, R. & Mangge, H. (2011) High density lipoprotein cholesterol level is a robust predictor of lipid peroxidation irrespective of gender, age, obesity, and inflammatory or metabolic biomarkers. *Clinica Chimica Acta* , in press.

4

Embryoprotective Therapy of Infertile Women with Polycystic Ovary Syndrome

Robert Hudeček and Renata Krajčovičová
Dept. Obstetrics and Gynecology, Masaryk University and University Hospital, Brno
Czech Republic

1. Introduction

1.1 Definition of infertility and habitual abortion

Infertility is defined as an inability of a woman to carry a pregnancy to a viable foetus. From the perspective of differential diagnosis, infertility differs from sterility, i.e. an inability of a woman to get pregnant. If a woman miscarries on at least three consecutive occasions, this is termed habitual abortion (or habitual pregnancy loss, HPL). Habitual abortion is a stand-alone nosological unit rather than an accumulation of circumstantial factors, as is confirmed by the lower incidence of foetal chromosomal aberrations in repeatedly miscarrying women compared to spontaneous abortions and a greater involvement of peristatic factors. A loss of all consecutive pregnancies in the first or second trimester is termed primary recurrent miscarriage. Secondary recurrent miscarriage is a situation when repeated miscarriages are preceded by a pregnancy leading to childbirth or an induced abortion. The term dysfertility is used if a woman miscarries on two consecutive occasions only (Zwinger, 2004).

1.2 Epidemiology and etiology of habitual abortion

Habitual abortion occurs in 1% of women in reproductive age and 15-38% of pregnancies result in spontaneous abortion. This number is, nevertheless, likely to be much higher as more than 40% of conceptions end before pregnancy is diagnosed (Madar, 2002). The frequency of spontaneous abortions increases with mother's age. Up to 90% of the first spontaneous abortions result from, usually de novo, chromosomal aneuploidy, whereas the risk of recurrence of the same abnormality is minimal (Roztočil, 2001). Causes of habitual abortion include age, anatomy factors, genetic factors, haematology factors, endocrine factors, infections, immunology factors, environmental factors, psychological factors, idiopathic factors.

1.3 Prerequisites of successful treatment of habitual abortion

Successful therapy of infertile women is subject to a careful and individualised differential diagnosis of habitual abortions. Comprehensive evaluation aimed at identification of the specific cause of infertility should be performed in the pregnant women who have previously repeatedly lost their pregnancy. Rigorous approach to diagnose the causes of repeated miscarriage is essential when an effective therapy is to be selected. Causal therapy of habitual pregnancy loss includes conservative pharmacological treatment, surgery and lifestyle changes.

2. Endocrine causes of recurrent pregnancy losses

An endocrinopathy is a common and severe cause of infertility. These are either gynaecology-related endocrinopathies and gynaecology-unrelated endocrinopathies. Gynaecology-related endocrinopathies results from ovarian hypofunction. Abnormal follicle stimulating/luteinizing hormone (FSH/LH) ratio and hyperandrogenism in the polycystic ovary syndrome are also considered as factors associated with an increased risk of habitual abortions. The proportion of first trimester miscarriages in women with the polycystic ovary syndrome is about 30–50% higher than in healthy women (Kauffman, 2003)

Gynaecology-unrelated endocrinopathies with unequivocal impact on fertility include thyreotoxicosis, hypothyreosis, diabetes mellitus, hyperprolactinaemia and obesity (Krajčovičová, 2007).

2.1 Gynaecology-related endocrinopathies

Epidemiologically, polycystic ovary syndrome is a highly prevalent gynaecology-related endocrinopathy. However, it is not solely a gynaecological condition but rather a disease with a range of metabolic and endocrine findings, including diabetes (Moller, 1993, Toscano, 1998). Ovarian hypofunction as a cause of habitual miscarriages represents another separate nosological unit of endocrinopathies with an impact on female reproductive function.

2.1.1 Polycystic ovary syndrome

It is estimated that polycystic ovary syndrome affects 5 - 10% of women of childbearing potential, with 35 - 45% of polycystic ovary syndrome patients being obese (Svačina, 2001). The real incidence of this syndrome in the population depends on the diagnostic criteria used and is probably higher than that published in the literature. Complications of pregnancy associated with maternal PCOS include increased prevalence of early pregnancy loss (EPL), gestational diabetes (GDM), pregnancy-induced hypertensive disorders (PET/PIH), and the birth of small-for-gestational-age (SGA) babies. Increased risk of EPL has been attributed to obesity, hyperinsulinaemia, elevated luteinizing hormone concentrations, and endometrial dysfunction. Avoiding obesity before pregnancy and treatment with metformin are therapeutic options, also for the increased prevalence of GDM (Homburg, 2006). Administration of metformin throughout pregnancy is a contentious issue. Screening pregnant women with PCOS for GDM and PET/PIH-especially if they are obese-is recommended, although data for a firm association between PCOS and PET/PIH is weak. Impaired insulin-mediated growth and foetal programming are possible explanations for a higher prevalence of SGA infants in mothers with PCOS (Homburg, 2006).

2.1.1.1 Polycystic ovary syndrome - pathophysiology

The mechanism behind metabolic and hormonal disposition for polycystic ovary syndrome, or what the primary disorder is, is rather unclear. Over the recent years, large groups of researchers have been involved in polycystic ovary syndrome research but the results are often controversial and confusing. Insulin resistance and the status of insulin receptors have frequently been investigated. Page: 3 Higher insulin independent autophosphorylation of insulin receptor at serine residue was observed. The role of IRS substrate disorders is also discussed as is the role of TNF-a, e.g. IRS-1 phosphorylation induced by TNF-a (Svačina, 2001). Defects of the glycoprotein PC-1 are being considered as another potential factor. Insulin resistance in male relatives has recently been shown. Phosphorylation of serine is a process that explains hyperanadrogenism as well as insulin resistance. This is a key process of androgen secretion in an ovary and adrenal glands and there also is important serine phosphorylation on insulin receptors (Svačina, 2001).

A number of studies focused on the clear association with abdominal obesity (even though some of the patients are not particularly obese) and it seems that it is only the women with higher abdominal fat that are insulin resistant and hyperandrogenemic. SHBG reduction is typical, particularly in obese patients. Sex hormone-binding globulin (SHBG) is the primary plasma transport protein for sex steroid hormones and regulates the bioavailability of these hormones to target tissues. The gene encoding SHBG is complex and any of several polymorphisms in SHBG have been associated with alterations in circulating SHBG levels (Chen, 2010). Epidemiological studies have revealed that low plasma SHBG levels are an early indicator of insulin resistance and predict the development of type 2 diabetes mellitus (T2DM) in both men and women. Although association between low SHBG levels and risk of diabetes could be explained by the observation that elevations in insulin suppress hepatic SHBG production. Recent studies documenting that the SHBG-altering polymorphisms are associated with risk of T2DM suggest that SHBG may have a more direct physiologic role in glucose homeostasis (Chen, 2010). However, the exact mechanism(s) underlying this association is not known (Chen, 2010). Non-diabetic women with the polycystic ovary syndrome (PCOS), a common endocrine disorder that is associated with insulin resistance, similarly demonstrate lower levels of SHBG. In light of studies investigating polymorphisms in SHBG and T2DM, our group and others have hypothesized that SHBG may represent a candidate gene for PCOS. In this manuscript, we review studies investigating the association between SHBG polymorphisms and PCOS. In summary, multiple studies in women with PCOS confirm that certain genetic polymorphisms are associated with circulating SHBG levels, but they are not consistently associated with PCOS per se. (Chen, 2010)

According to some authors, insulin resistance can be found in women with anovulation cycles only. Women with polycystic ovary syndrome have lower basal energy expenditure as well as postprandial termogenesis. This is an analogy with android obesity, metabolic syndrome and diabetes. A relative lack of gestagens and, consequently, dominance of cortisol on receptors in abdominal fat may also contribute to the pathogenesis. This results in higher level of free fatty acids and insulin resistance.

To assess the diabetes risk score in polycystic ovary syndrome (PCOS) and in different phenotypes of PCOS and controls was observed and evaluated by overweight premenopausal women with PCOS, non PCOS or controls folowing factors: Finnish Diabetes Risk Score, anthropometrics, oral glucose tolerance test (OGTT), glucose, insulin, and reproductive hormone levels. The women with PCOS had higher adiposity, abdominal adiposity and 120-minute OGTT glucose. The women with PCOS and non-PCOS had elevated 120-minute OGTT insulin compared with controls. The women with PCOS and non-PCOS had similar diabetes risk scores, but both had higher diabetes risk score compared with controls after matching age and BMI. The women with PCOS (4%) and non-PCOS (12%) had a lower prevalence of low risk of diabetes scores compared with controls

(50%) and they have similar Finnish Diabetes Risk Scores and elevated scores relative to controls independent of age and adiposity. Similar clinical screening and treatment practices for type 2 diabetes are warranted for both phenotypes of PCOS (Moran, 2011)

Another research study compared pregnancy outcome, specifically the prevalence of gestational diabetes mellitus (GDM), in a group of patients with polycystic ovary syndrome (PCOS) to a group of healthy weight-matched women. Pregnancies of women with PCOS, who had been treated for infertility were compared with a group of age- and weight-matched controls. There were no significant differences in the prevalence of pregnancy complications such as gestational diabetes mellitus, pregnancy-induced hypertension (PIH) and premature deliveries between the group of PCOS patients and the controls. When differences in age and weight between PCOS patients and controls are negligible, PCOS is not associated with a higher risk of pregnancy complications. (Hašková, 2003)

2.1.1.2 Polycystic ovary syndrome - diagnosis

The international conference in Bethesda in 1990 have recommended three diagnostic criteria: hyperandrogenism, chronic anovulation (enzyme deficits at a level of adrenal glands, e.g. 21-hydroxylase deficit as well as hyperprolactinaemia and androgen-producing tumours should be excluded) and hyperinsulinmia (Svačina, 2001). Frequent, although not exclusive, symptoms include hirsutism, alopecia and acne. There may be no morphological changes on the ovaries. An older definition assumed the presence of at least eight subcapsular cysts in the ovaries of 10 cm in diameter. Higher LH/FSH ratio (usually above 2,0), previous important endocrine diagnostic criterion, is not anymore required for the diagnosis (Toscano, 1998).

2.1.1.3 Polycystic ovary syndrome – treatment

Management of polycystic ovary syndrome (PCOS) usually spans woman's reproductive years. While treatment of androgenic symptoms is often a primary concern, periodically, the regimen has to be modified because of a desire for pregnancy. At this time the couple should be evaluated for factors that may contribute to infertility and this should include semen analysis. However, for many, anovulation is likely to be the cause of infertility and ovulation induction is generally required. The premise on which ovulation induction in PCOS is based is two-fold: increasing ovarian exposure to follicle stimulating hormone (FSH) and/or correcting hormonal derangements. Potential differences in pathogenesis, evidenced clinically by phenotypic diversity, would suggest that treatment should be individualized. These options include the use of clomiphene citrate, insulin sensitizers, and the combination. Protocols for ovulation induction with FSH injections are outlined and the relative risks of multiple gestation and severe ovarian hyperstimulation syndrome. The use of aromatase inhibitors and the occasional use of glucocorticoids are briefly reviewed, and indications for in vitro fertilization and laparoscopic ovarian diathermy outlined (Nader, 2010).

2.1.1.3.1 Clomiphene citrate and insulin sensitizers

The knowledge on the role of insulin resistance in the pathogenesis of PCOS has led to the use of insulin sensitizers in PCOS treatment. Metformin was the first to be used in 1994. Administration of metformin results in decreased androgen and LH levels, improvement in insulin sensitivity and normalization of menstrual cycle (Legro, 2007). Metformin decreases liver gluconeogenesis and reduces oxidation of free fatty acids. It increases uptake of glucose by skeletal muscles and fat tissue, improves dyslipidemia and it has other specific effects in the ovaries (Mansfield, 2003). Metformin impacts on ovarian steroidogenesis by reducing androgen production, improving the adverse environment of the endometrium and improves ovarian function. It seems so far that metformin (and glitazones) has no or insignificantly positive effect on hirsutism (Šarapatková, 2008). A meta-analysis of metformin studies showed that, compared to placebo, metformin significantly increases the occurrence of ovulation (Lord, 2003). However, it is not clear yet whether treating women with PCOS and with normal BMI and insulin sensitivity with metformin is beneficial. Also, there is a question whether clomiphene should be used alone or in combination with metformin or whether metformin monotherapy should be used to enable infertile women with PCOS to become pregnant and deliver a healthy baby. In a 6-month study comparing all three approaches, clomiphene led to the highest pregnancy and live birth rates. Addition of metformin to therapy in this study did not show a significant advantage over clomiphene monotherapy. However, possible positive effect of this combination cannot be excluded. Induction of ovulation itself does not mean higher likelihood of conceiving and giving birth to a healthy child. Metformin provided, in line with previous findings, an improvement in parameters of insulin sensitivity, BMI, insulin and proinsulin levels, while insulin resistance and testosterone levels declined. Nevertheless, these effects may not be associated with higher rate of live births (Legro, 2007).

Recently, glitazones, other insulin resistance modifying agents, have been tested in women with PCOS. They improve the effects of insulin in the liver, skeletal muscles and fat tissue. Similar to metformin, they also directly impact on ovarian steroidogenesis (Mansfield, 2003). Decrease in insulin levels results in decline in the levels of circulating androgens. Glitazones also reduce the levels of plasminogen activator inhibitor-1. Glitazones are not widely used in clinical practice and they are contraindicated in pregnancy (Šarapatková, 2008). The use of metformin in patients diagnosed with hyperinsulinaemia and in women with the polycystic ovary syndrome represents a therapeutic use of an insulin sensitizer with promising effects in anovulation sterility and dysfertility.

2.1.1.3.2 Protocols for ovulation induction with FSH and in vitro fertilisation

Women with PCOS and a history of habitual abortions or a history of sterility due to anovulation frequently undergo IVF cycles requiring ovarian stimulation with follicle-stimulating hormone (FSH). In his retrospective study, Kdous compared standard long GnRH agonist protocol (Triptolerin) and GnRH antagonist regimens (Cetrorelix) in polycystic ovary syndrome (PCOS) patients undergoing controlled ovarian stimulation (COS) for ICSI cycles. He found that GnRH antagonist protocol is a short and simple protocol with a significant reduction in the incidence of OHSS and gonadotropin levels. However, GnRH antagonist protocol provides a lower live birth rate and an increased risk of early pregnancy loss compared to the GnRH agonist long protocol (Kdous 2009). Well-established micromanipulation techniques, the ICSI and PICSI methods, are successfully used for IVF in women with PCOS. Ovarian hyperstimulation syndrome (OHSS) is a feared complication of IVF. Women with PCOS are at a greater risk of developing OHSS because of the higher number of follicles produced in the ovaries following FSH stimulation (Moosová, 2011).

2.1.1.3.3 Aromatase inhibitors

Aromatase inhibitors block the final step in the enzymatic estrogen production: aromatization of the A-cycle of aromatizable androgens, specifically androstendione and testosteron. Substances interfering with aromatase activity have been available for many years. However, the substances used during the aminoglutethimide era were non-specific and had a poor safety profile. The third generations of aromatase inhibitors are highly specific and virtually free of adverse events. These substances are licensed for treatment of breast cancer in postmenopausal women with advanced disease or as adjuvant treatment. Temporary inhibition of estradiol production in women with active ovaries leads to increased gonadotropin concentrations and, consequently, stimulation of follicle growth. This is undesirable in patients with ovarian cancer and thus aromatase inhibitors are not used in premenopausal women unless the production of gonadotropins is blocked. On the other hand, this effect is highly desirable in infertile women. Aromatase inhibitors may be used in women who do not ovulate but their no meaning (PCOS-type oligo-ovulation) or in ovulating women in whom higher number of follicles are required (idiopathic infertility, age factor, or prior to IVF). Preliminary studies published thus far show rather convincingly that aromatase inhibitors are effective in inducing ovulation in infertile women (Mitwally, 2006). Letrozole (one of aromatase inhibitors), though reported to be an effective ovulation inducing agent, warrants larger randomized trials. The purpose of this study is to compare the efficacy of letrozole with that of rFSH and clomiphene citrate (CC)/rFSH for ovarian stimulation in IUI cycles. In randomized, prospective, single-blinded clinical trial. 1387 PCOS women after CC failure were randomized into three groups: Group A received letrozole, Group B received CC with two doses rFSH and Group C received continuous rFSH day 2 onwards until hCG injection. RESULTS: Group A, B and C had an ovulation rate of 79.30%, 56.95% and 89.89% and cycle cancellation rate of 20.70%, 43.05% and 10.11%, respectively. Pregnancy rates in Group A, B and C were 23.39%, 14.35% and 17.92%, while the miscarriage rates were 13.80%, 16.67% and 14.52%, respectively. CONCLUSION: Letrozole appears to be a suitable ovulation inducing agent in PCOS women with CC failure and is found to be most effective when baseline estradiol level >60 pg/ml. (Ganesh, 2009).

2.1.1.3.4 Glucocorticoids

In recurrently miscarrying women with PCOS, the presence of high titres of antizonal and antisperm antibodies should be excluded and potential insufficiency of sperm cell head's enzymatic status considered. Patients in whom implantation is a problem, the presence of antizonal and antiendometrial antibodies has to be excluded. High levels of antiphospholipid antibodies and other mechanisms aimed at immunological mother-semi-allogeneic graft tolerance might adversely affect the entire IVF process. Therapy is often carefully selected with respect to a patient's age, character and type of antibodies and the number of IVF cycles. Most frequently, micromanipulation is combined with temporary immunosuppression (short-term administration of glucocorticoids, e.g. Prednison 5mg dosed 1-1/2-0 daily) and long-term antioxidant treatment (Ulčová-Gallová, 2001).

2.1.1.3.5 Treatment by laparoscopic ovarian diathermy

Laparoscopic ovarian drilling is used as one of the options for surgical management of infertility in patients with polycystic ovary syndrome. This method is performed as laparoscopic electrocautery with monopolar needle. Ovarian surface is systematically perforated with a needle and the surgery is frequently combined with a test of tubal patency or hysteroscopy as part of a comprehensive diagnostic laparoscopy. The effect of drilling on reproductive function was evaluated by a number of studies. Kong compared the effects of laparoscopic ovarian drilling in treating infertile polycystic ovarian syndrome in patients with and without metabolic syndrome. A total of 89 infertile anovulatory polycystic ovarian syndrome patients, who underwent laparoscopic ovarian drilling with completed metabolic screening and seen over a 5-year period. The main outcome measures were clinical, hormonal and metabolic characteristics, as well as spontaneous ovulation rates, reproductive outcomes, and a risk of gestational diabetes after laparoscopic ovarian drilling. Approximately one fifth (21%) of polycystic ovary syndrome patients had metabolic syndrome. There were no differences in spontaneous ovulation rates (68% vs 61%, P=0.76), cumulative pregnancy rates (68% vs 61%, P=0.77), and a risk of gestational diabetes (64% vs 42%, P=0.13) between patients with and without metabolic syndrome. Laparoscopic ovarian drilling was equally effective in inducing ovulation in polycystic ovary syndrome patients with metabolic syndrome. Thus, patients with metabolic syndrome should not be excluded from laparoscopic ovarian drilling, which has an additional advantage of enabling concurrent full tubo-peritoneal assessment (Kong, 2010).

In randomized double-blind placebo-controlled pilot study Nasr evaluated N-acetyl-cysteine (NAC) as an adjunctive therapy following unilateral laparoscopic ovarian drilling (LOD) for clomiphene citrate-resistant women with polycystic ovary syndrome (PCOS). Patients with clomiphene citrate-resistant PCOS who underwent unilateral LOD were assigned randomly to receive either NAC 1.2 g/d or placebo for 5 days starting at day 3 of the cycle for 12 consecutive cycles. The primary outcome was pregnancy rate; secondary outcomes were ovulation rates, endometrial thickness and pregnancy outcome. Baseline clinical, endocrine, and sonographic characteristics were similar in the two groups. A significant increase in both ovulation and pregnancy rates was observed in the NAC group, compared with placebo [87% versus 67% (RR 1.3; 95% CI 1.2-2.7) and 77% versus 57% (RR 1.4; 95% CI 1.1-2.7), respectively, P<0.01]. Moreover, miscarriage rates were significantly lower and live birth rates were significantly higher in the NAC group [8.7% versus 23.5% (RR 0.4; 95% CI 0.1-3.7) and 67% versus 40% (RR 1.7; 95% CI 0.3-3.5), respectively, P<0.01]. NAC, a novel adjuvant therapy to be used following unilateral LOD, might improve overall reproductive outcome (Nasr, 2010).

2.1.2 Ovarian hypofunction

The main therapeutic aim of ovarian hypofunction management is to treat fertility disorders and to substitute the lacking hormones. Treatment of ovarian hypofunction-related dysfertility by assisted reproduction methods represents a complex issue. This group of patients ("low responders") typically presents with low ovarian response to stimulation of foliculogenesis in *in vitro* fertilization cycles.

2.1.2.1 Ovarian hypofunction - pathophysiology

When discussing causes of recurrent miscarriages, experts differ in their opinion on the role of luteal insufficiency, the so called implantation factor. This is when a discrepancy occurs between adequate endometrial secretion and high nutritional needs of the fertilized egg, either during its free transport through the uterus before implantation or during histiotrophic nutrition. This discrepancy may lead to a suppression of embryonic development and the pregnancy ends in miscarriage in the first trimester (Erlebacher, 2004).

2.1.2.2 Ovarian hypofunction - diagnosis

During a pre-conception assessment, luteal insufficiency should be considered in patients with very short secretory phase by basal temperature readings, recurrent severe retardation of secretory transformation of the endometrium by microabrasion, or a significant reduction in serum progesterone in the secretory phase of the menstrual cycle (Zwinger, 2004).

2.1.2.3 Ovarian hypofunction - treatmen

No optimal, universal and adequately effective IVF stimulation protocol can be found in the literature (Mardesic, 1995). In these stimulation cycles, higher doses of gonadotropic hormones are usually used and a lower number of oocytes are obtained. Whilst fertilization rate is within the norm, there is significantly lower percentage of obtained clinical pregnancies. With higher incidence of early pregnancy losses (mainly in women above 40 years of age), the percentage of pregnancies ending in a delivery of a healthy foetus in women with reduced ovarian reserve is significantly lower than in dysfertile couples with other than ovarian factors of infertility.

Stimulation protocols in this group of patients should use higher doses of rFSH (max. 300 IU/D), in combination with GnRH antagonists (from 6th DC). Follicular phase of the cycle should not be prolonged because of the risk of premature ovulation and ovulation should be induced by an administration of 10 000 IU hCG when a minimum of 3 follicles ≥ 17mm are visible by UZ folliculometry. Oocytes should be withdrawn no later than 16th day of a menstrual cycle. Embryos obtained through prolonged cultivation and assisted hatching should be transferred under gestagen facilitation of luteal phase no longer than 20th DC. The most reliable and most successful method of achieving pregnancy in POF women is *in vitro* fertilization using a donated oocyte together with oestrogen-gestagen preparation of the endometrium (Hudeček, 2004). Stimulation of ovulation with gonadotropins in women with POF is ineffective. Centres of assisted reproduction report pregnancy rate in women with POF around 40 - 50% per cycle. Even though the child is genetically related to the father only, not to the mother, this method of infertility treatment in women with POF is generally acceptable, especially because the woman has a chance to carry the pregnancy to term herself and is able to breast feed the child (Žáková, 2006). There is about 5% chance in women who do not accept donated oocytes that they are able to get spontaneously pregnant despite the diagnosis of POF. The likelihood of this depends mainly on aetiology of POF (Altchek, 2003).

There are discussions in the literature on utilization of native IVF cycles, protocols with minimum stimulation, including a possibility to convert a stimulation cycle into intrauterine insemination (Shahine, 2009, Schimberni, 2009). Even though these techniques of assisted reproduction show significantly lower efficacy, they may be considered as a treatment option in individual specific cases.

A long-term hormonal therapy leading to pseudopregnancy followed by an administration of gestagens during a subsequent pregnancy (usually during the first trimester) is indicated in patients with luteal insufficiency. Decrease in estrogen receptors as progesterone receptor promoters can be modulated by the means of gestagen substitution (supra-physiological doses of progesterone - 150 mg per day) (Hudeček, 2004).

2.2 Gynaecology-unrelated endocrinopathies

2.2.1 Thyrotoxicosis

Thyrotoxicosis (hyperthyreosis) is a clinical syndrome caused by an overproduction of thyroid hormones. The main signs and symptoms of thyrotoxicosis result from hypermetabolism due to intensified oxidative processes in the body caused by excessive concentrations of these hormones. Graves-Basedow disease is the most frequent form of hyperthyreosis (60-85% of thyrotoxicoses) with a production of anti-thyroid peroxidase autoantibodies and anti-thyrotropin receptor antibodies. Approximately 10 - 30% of hyperthyreoses involve toxic multinodular goitre with autoimmune production of thyroid hormones (T3, T4). Inflammations also frequently cause hyperthyreosis by provoking T3 and T4 secretion (Ďuriš, 2001).

Clinical signs of thyrotoxicosis include nervousness, hand tremor, weight loss with increased appetite, palpitations, heat intolerance and hyperhidrosis. Other subjective symptoms include emotional lability, muscle weakness and diarrhoea.

Objective symptoms include tachycardia or atrial fibrillation, high pulse pressure (the difference between systolic and diastolic pressure), precordial pulsation, and accentuated first sound above the apex of the heart. Gynaecological symptoms include polymenorrhoea, metrorrhagia, sometimes amenorrhoea or sterility. Warm, soft skin, goitre and increased psychomotor reactivity or restlessness may all contribute to the complete clinical picture of hyperthyreosis.

2.2.1.1 Pathophysiology of thyrotoxicosis

Hyperthyreosis might be accompanied by an increased level of gonadotropins, SHBG, estrogens and androgens (although the free fraction of these steroids is lowered due to the increased SHBG levels). A change to the concentration of free steroids and direct effect of thyroid hormones frequently causes anovulation and luteal insufficiency. Hyperthyreosis might be associated with polymenorrhoea and metrorrhagia as well as amenorrhoea and sterility. Some studies have shown that the autoimmune thyroiditis (AT) itself, without obvious or subclinical thyroid gland dysfunction, diagnosed before conception, is associated with infertility, recurring miscarriages and more frequent failure of assisted reproduction methods (Stagnaro-Green , 2004, Poppe 2003).

One theory uses immunological mechanisms to explain the association between infertility and AT without thyroid gland dysfunction (Poppe, 2003). Some published papers identified concurrent occurrence of anti-thyroid and anti-ovarian antibodies; this may contribute to explain the association between AT and ovarian dysfunction (Sterlz, 1997). However, cell immunity is more likely to be responsible for recurring miscarriages. According to this theory, AT is one of the symptoms of a systemic autoimmune disease and represents an indicator of an alteration of the woman's immune system responsible for recurring miscarriages. Elevated levels of CD 5/20 lymphocytes identified in women with AT and an increased risk of miscarriage supports this theory (Roberts, 1996).

2.2.1.2 Diagnosis of thyrotoxicosis

Thyrotoxicosis is diagnosed from the patient's medical history and an assessment of the clinical picture and laboratory parameters. Thyrotoxicosis is characterised by decreased and even undetectable TSH level and hyperthyroxinemia. TSH levels above 0.1 mU/L exclude a significant form of thyrotoxicosis. An optimal way of treatment should be decided from serum autoantibody levels (anti-thyroid peroxidase autoantibodies, anti-thyrotropin receptor antibodies). Imaging methods and gammagraphy of the thyroid gland are also important (Ďuriš, 2001).

2.2.1.3 Treatment of thyrotoxicosis

Treatment of hyperthyreosis includes lifestyle changes (regular, substantial food intake, avoiding extreme temperatures and excessive physical activity), thyreostatic treatment, subtotal strumectomy and treatment with radioiodine. Pharmacological thyreostatic treatment suppresses the overproduction of thyroid hormones by the thyroid gland. The thiouracil derivatives and carbimazole represent the first line treatment. A surgical treatment, subtotal strumectomy, can be applied when remission was achieved using a thyrostatic agent (florid thyrotoxicosis is a contraindication to any surgery as the patient is at risk of developing thyrotoxic crisis). An administration of a therapeutic dose of radioiodine is indicated when thyrotoxicosis is a co-morbidity to cardiopathy and when thyrotoxicosis recurred following strumectomy (Ďuriš, 2001).

2.2.2 Hypothyreosis

Hypothyreosis is a disorder characterized by decreased thyroid hormone levels. The prevalence of hypothyreosis in the population is about 5-8%, higher in women than men (8:1) and increases with age. Hypothyreosis should always be thought of in older women (prevalence 15 - 20%), not only if the patient presents with specific symptoms but also if they report general complaints such as fatigue, depression and myalgia. Autoimmune thyroid gland disease as well as, understandably, post-thyroidectomy states or treatment with radioiodine are among the most frequent causes. The clinical picture is diverse and includes fatigue, inefficiency, somnolence, depression, poor cold tolerance, weight gain, feeling of pressure on the neck (may also occur if the thyroid gland is not enlarged during AIT), dry skin, myalgia and arthralgia.

The thyroid gland may be enlarged, nodular as well as reduced, thinking and motor functions are slowed down, hypomimia, oedema of the face, eye lid oedema, macroglosy, deep voice. Anaemia is usually normochromic, pernicious in about 10% of cases and associated with autoimmunity, gynaecological symptoms include menstrual cycle disorders, menorrhagia, infertility and galactorrhoea (Brunová, 2008).

2.2.2.1 Pathophysiology of hypothyreosis

Hypothyreosis is one of the most important endocrine primarily non-gyneacological endocrinopaties that affect female fertility. Untreated hypothyreosis reduces fertility, increases the incidence of spontaneous abortions and increases the incidence of premature deliveries (Ďuriš, 2001). Manifest hypothyreosis is frequently linked to anovulation, oligomenorrhoea or amenorrhoea and infertility. Thyroid hormones directly impact on the correct function of oocytes, lutein cells and granulosa cells. In addition, hypothyreosis is associated with a reduction of gonadotropins (particularly the luteinizing hormone) and with an increase in prolactin levels; this results in a decreased production of ovarian steroids. Reduced levels of thyroid hormones result in their reduced production and, consequently, the sex hormone binding globulin (SHBG) levels also decline, the level of free testosterone increases as does peripheral aromatization of androstendione to estrone (Krassas, 2000). Thyroid hormones are very important for intrauterine foetal development, particularly for the development of the brain and for the development of the hypothalamic-pituitary-thyroid axis. Gravidity represents a period when an increased production of thyroid hormones is required. The foetus depends completely on the mother during the first trimester, and the contribution of the mother to foetal hormonal levels remains significant throughout (maternal productions after birth represent about 30% of thyroxin in the umbilical cord blood) and its importance increases during foetal thyreopathies and insufficient production of thyroid hormones by the foetus. Total production of thyroid hormones in gravidity increases by about 25 - 30% (Karásek, 2007). A tendency to subclinical hypothyreosis during pregnancy was observed in a significant proportion of women with normal free thyroxin and TSH levels. The impact of subclinical or even manifest hypothyreosis during pregnancy on recurrent miscarriages is evidenced by the time when miscarriages occur - usually during the first trimester when the foetus is completely dependent on its mother's production of thyroid hormones (Poppe, 2003).

2.2.2.2 Diagnosis of hypothyreosis

Primary hypothyreosis by increased TSH levels and reduced free T3 and free T4 levels, central hypothyreosis is then characterized by decreased or normal (i.e. not adequately increased) TSH levels (Brunová, 2008).

2.2.2.3 Treatment of hypothyreosis

Treatment of hypothyreosis is initiated with small doses of 25 µg/day and sometimes just 12.5 µg/day of thyroxin. The dose is increased every 7 - 14 days to the expected maintenance dose. The dose is reduced again if the patient poorly tolerates the treatment, i.e. suffers from palpitations, angina pectoris or has signs of heart failure. The demand for thyroid hormone secretion increases during pregnancy and thus thyroxin dose in mothers previously treated for hypothyreosis should be increased during pregnancy by 30% or even 50% (Brunová, 2008).

2.2.3 Diabetes mellitus

Diabetes mellitus is a group of metabolic diseases characterized by chronic hyperglycaemia developing as a result of insulin secretion disorder or as an effect of insulin or a combination of these factors. The main symptom is hyperglycaemia. From biochemical perspective, diabetes influences metabolism of carbohydrates, lipids and proteins. Clinically, it is responsible for the development of microvascular and macrovascular complications associated with organ specific degenerative processes and leading to neuropathic complications (diabetic ketoacidosis, cardiovascular complications, diabetic retinopathy, neuropathy, nephropathy), (Ďuriš, 2001).

Classification of diabetes mellitus:

a. Diabetes mellitus
   1. Type 1 diabetes mellitus - insulin-dependent
   2. Type 2 diabetes mellitus - non-insulin-dependent
   3. Malnutrition-related diabetes mellitus
   4. Other specific types (secondary) of diabetes mellitus – hyperglycaemia associated with another cause (e.g. pancreatic disease, endocrinopathy).

b. Impaired glucose tolerance
c. Gestational diabetes mellitus

2.2.3.1 Pathophysiology of diabetes mellitus

Diabetic female patients are more frequently diagnosed with an ovulatory disorder leading to infertility. A comparison of hormonal profile of diabetic patients suffering from amenorrhoea and women with regular menses suggests different pathophysiological mechanisms, specifically the presence of hyperandrogenism. The effects of hyperinsulinaemia are particularly important. Hyperinsulinaemia stimulates androgenesis in the ovaries. This stimulation is via IGF receptors found in the ovaries present in sufficient amount. This is either a traditional example of the linkage between insulin and steroidogenesis or a hyperreactivity of ovarian receptors for a different reason (Svačina, 1997). According to this theory, changes to pituitary hormones might be secondary, determined by higher level of androgens. Defect of serine phosphorylation with a common manifestation on peripheral insulin receptors, ovaries and adrenal glands represents another significant theory. A slight increase in total testosterone and androstendione levels occur despite concurrent increase in catabolism of androgens. Under normal circumstances, around 66% of the circulating testosterone is bound to the *sex-hormone-binding globulin* (SHBG). When fasting (e.g. anorexia), SHBG concentration increases. On the contrary, SHBG level decreases with increasing BMI, mainly in android obesity and polycystic ovary syndrome (particularly if associated with obesity) and in association with diabetes mellitus; this further increases android hormone concentrations. Hyperinsulinism that is associated with this disease, is one of the possible explanations. Experimental *in vitro* studies show that insulin has an inhibitory effect on SHBG synthesis in the liver (Cogswel, 2001).

Hyperinsulinaemia is diagnosed in as many as 27% of women with a history of habitual abortion (Carrington, 2005) Hyperinsulinaemia influences endometrial functions by reducing the levels of the two main endometrial hormones, glycodelin and IGFBP (insulin-like growth factor binding protein). Hyperinsulinaemia is diagnosed in 40–50% of women with the polycystic ovary syndrome (Kauffman, 2003).

Spontaneous abortion is seen more often in women with decompensated diabetes mellitus (DM) during early pregnancy. It is more frequent in poorly compensated type 1 DM patients, although it is sometimes diagnosed in patients with type 2 DM that had not been diagnosed prior to their pregnancy. Pregnancy is considered a diabetogenic state and the onset of gestational diabetes mellitus is associated with an increased insulin resistance (Hájek, 2004).

Decompensated type 1 diabetic females suffer more frequently from spontaneous abortions (even repeatedly), particularly as a consequence of higher incidence of diabetic embryopathy DE (2-3x more frequent in diabetics in comparison to healthy population). Diabetic embryopathy is a congenital developmental defect or a malformation of the foetus not compatible with life. Etiopathogenesis of DE has not been elucidated yet. Clinical and experimental knowledge confirm that hyperglycaemia is the main metabolic teratogen. Direct link between HbA1c level at the beginning of pregnancy and the incidence of diabetic embryopathy has been confirmed (Ďuriš, 2001).

2.2.3.2 Diagnosis of diabetes mellitus

Diagnosis of diabetes mellitus is made from patient's urine glucose levels and blood testing with oral Glucose Tolerance Testing (oGTT). Prior to conception, current metabolic compensation - glycaemic profile, glycosylated haemoglobin (HbA1C) and diabetic complications assessment - is reviewed. Pregnancy is not recommended in women with severe diabetic organ complications (Hájek, 2004)

2.2.3.3 Treatment of diabetes mellitus

Treatment should focus on supplementing or inhibiting the effects of the relevant hormones and careful diabetes mellitus control (dietary regimen, insulinotherapy).

Classification of DM therapies:

1. Non-pharmacological therapy
   - Patient education
   - Diet
   - Physical activity
2. Pharmacological treatment
   - Insulin (in insulin-dependent type 1 DM and always during pregnancy with any type of diabetes)
   - Oral antidiabetics (non-insulin dependent type 2 DM)

Treatment should be comprehensive, managed by an experienced diabetologist (Ďuriš, 2001). Prescribing metformin, an insulin sensitizer, in women with PCOS represents therapeutic application of an agent with promising effects in the area of anovulation sterility and dysfertility (Višňová, 2003).

2.2.4 Hyperprolactinaemia

Prolactin is a polypeptide hormone synthesised by lactotropic cells of the anterior pituitary. The main effect of this hormone is ensuring adequate postpartum lactation. In collaboration with other hormones, prolactin influences the growth of mammary glands during pregnancy. Prolactin levels in women who do not breast feed decline quickly within two weeks after birth and ovulation is likely to restart within 10 weeks. Hyperprolactinaemia is a disease with a pathological increase in prolactin levels out of postpartum period (Ďuriš, 2001).

2.2.4.1 Pathophysiology of hyperprolactinaemia

Excessive prolactin levels reduce the effects of hypothalamic GnRH and thus normal pulsate secretion of luteinizing hormone and follicle-stimulating hormone. Elevated prolactin levels also have a negative effect on luteinizing hormone increase in the middle of a menstrual cycle (peak LH). Basal levels of gonadotropins are within the norm. Lack of pulsate gonadotropin secretion leads to the functional hypogonadism with anovulation. Anovulation cycles are clinically manifested as oligomenorrhoea or amenorrhoea with subsequent reduction in fertility. The clinical picture typically also includes galactorrhoea, symptoms of estrogen insufficiency (reduced vaginal secretion, osteoporosis), mood swings and hirsutism. Hyperprolactinaemia is found in women with chronic renal insufficiency, with liver cirrhosis and those using certain drugs (psychotropics, antiemetics, antihypertensives, H1 and H2 receptor antagonists). It is found in patients with hypothalamic disease (cranial and nasopharyngeal irradiation), pituitary disease (tumours - prolactinoma, metastases, meningioma), with primary hypothyreosis or it may be idiopathic (Ďuriš, 2001).

2.2.4.2 Diagnosis of hyperprolactinaemia

The diagnosis of hyperprolactinaemia is made from rigorous medical history, detailed clinical assessment and blood prolactin levels. Prolactin levels above 16 ng/mL are considered as hyperprolactinaemia. Levels exceeding 200 ng/mL suggest prolactinoma, 200 - 500 ng/mL is pathognomonic for prolactinoma and the levels exceeding 1000 ng/mL evidence an invasive tumour expanding to sinus cavernosum. Levels below 100 ng/mL are usually not a symptom of a pituitary tumour (Ďuriš, 2001).

2.2.4.3 Treatment of hyperprolactinaemia

Treatment of hyperprolactinaemia is determined by the primary cause. Surgery, specifically the transsphenoidal hypophysectomy (transcranial approach is required when large macroprolactinomas are treated), is the method of choice for diagnosed microprolactinomas and macroprolactinomas. Radiation therapy is a complementary method in patients with incurable microprolactinomas. Pharmacological treatment is used in patients with hyperprolactinaemia caused by hypothalamo-pituitary dysfunction or in those with idiopathic hyperprolactinaemia. Pharmacological agents used include dopamine agonists that normalize prolactin secretion in about 85 - 90% of patients and reduce the tumour in about 50%. The most frequently used agents include ergoline derivatives bromocryptine, lisuride and terguride (Ďuriš, 2001).

3. Conclusion

A comprehensive and interdisciplinary approach is required to diagnose the causes of habitual miscarriage in a woman. The use of simple and widely available assessment methods in the basic differential diagnosis algorithm is preferred. If these do not provide a clear identification of aetiology of infertility, it is suitable to use more specific and technically demanding techniques. Adequate differential diagnosis enables determination of likely aetiology and a use of an appropriately targeted therapy.

4. References

Altchek, A., Deligdisch, L., Kase, N.,G. (2003). *Diagnosis and management of ovarian disorders.* ISBN 0120536420, New York, United States

Brunova, J. (2008). *Diagnostics and therapy of disorders thyroid function.* Med Pro Praxi, ISSN - 1214-8687, Olomouc, Czech Republic

Carrington, B., Sacks, G., Regan, L. et al. (2005). *Recurrent miscarriage: pathophysiology and outcome.* Obstet Gyn, ISSN 1040-872X, Washington, USA

Cogswell, ME. et al. (2001). *Obesity in women of childbearing age: risks, prevention and treatment.* Prim Care Update Ob/Gyn, ISSN: 1068-607X Elsevier, NewYork, USA

Ďuriš, I.; Hulín, I., Bernadič, M. et al. (2001). *Principles of internal medicine.* SAP, ISBN 80-88908-69-8, Bratislava, Slovakia

Erlebacher, A., Zhang, D., Parlow, AF. et al. (2004). *Ovarian insuficiency and early pregnancy loss.* T Jour of Clinic Invest, ISSN 00219738, New York, USA

Ganesh, A., Goswami, SK., Chattopadhyay, R., Chaudhury, K., Chakravarty, B. (2009). *Comparison of letrozole with continuous gonadotropins and clomiphene-gonadotropin combination for ovulation induction in 1387 PCOS women after clomiphene citrate failure: a randomized prospective clinical trial.* Journal of Assisted Reproduction & Genetics. PMCID: PMC2649330 Kharakpur, India

Hájek, Z. (2004). *High-risk and pathologic pregnancy.* Grada, ISBN 8024704188, Praha, Czech Republic

Haškova, L., Cibula, D., Rezabek, K., Hill, M., Fanta, M., Zivny, J. (2003). *Pregnancy outcome in women with PCOS and in controls matched by age and weight.* Human Reproduction, ISSN 1460-2350, Oxford, UK

Homburg, R. (2006). *Pregnancy complications in PCOS.* Best Practice & Research Clinical Endocrinology & Metabolism, ISSN 1521-690x Amsterdam, The Netherlands

Hudeček, R., Ventruba, P., Juránková, E. et al. (2004). *Therapeutic posibiliites of asisted reproduction at perimenopausal women.* Prakt Gyn, ISSN 1801-8750, Brno, Czech Republic

Chen, C., Smothers, J., Lange, A., Nestler, J E., Strauss, J F., Wickham, E P. (2010) *Sex hormone-binding globulin genetic variation: associations with type 2 diabetes mellitus and polycystic ovary syndrome.* Minerva Endocrinologica, ISSN 0391-1977, Shanghai, China

Kauffman, RP., Castracane, D., Kosasa, T. (2003). *Polycystic ovary syndrome.* Gynek po prom. ISSN 1213-2578, Praha, Czech Republic

Karásek, D.; Oborná, I.; Fryšták, Z (2007) *Autoimune thyreoiditis and sterility.* Int Med; 9(9): 394-397. ISSN - 1212-7299, Olomouc, Czech Republic

Kdous, M., Chaker, A., Bouyahia, M., Zhioua, F., Zhioua, A. (2009). *Increased risk of early pregnancy loss and lower live birth rate with GNRH antagonist vs. long GNRH agonist protocol in PCOS women undergoing controlled ovarian hyperstimulation.* Tunisie Medicale, ISSN 0041-4131, Hôpital Sadiki, Tunis

Kong, GW., Cheung, LP., Lok, IH. (2011). *Effects of laparoscopic ovarian drilling in treating infertile anovulatory polycystic ovarian syndrome patients with and without metabolic syndrome.* Medical Journal, ISSN 1024-2708, Hong Kong

Krajčovičová, R., Hudeček, R., Kalvodová, J. (2007). *Diferential diagnostics and treatment of habitual misscaries.* Prakt Gyn. ISSN 1801-8750, Brno, Czech Republic

Krassas, G.E. (2000). *Thyroid disease and female reproduction.* Fertil Steril, ISSN: 0015-0282, Thessaloniki, Greece

Legro, R., S., et al. (2007). *Clomiphene, metformin, or both for infertility in the polycystic ovary syndrome.* N Eng J Med, ISSN 0028-4793, Massachusets Medical Society, Boston

Lord, J.,M., Flight, I. Norman, R., J(2003). *Insulin-sensiting drugs (metformin, troglitazone, rosiglitazone,pioglitazone, D-chiro-inositol) for polycystic ovary syndrome.* Cochrane Database Syst Rev, CD003053.

Madar, J., Nouza, D., Nováková, D. (2002). *Imunological aspects of habitual misscaries.* Moderni gynekologie a porodnictví. ISSN 1211-1058, Praha , Czech Republic

Mansfield, R., Galea, R., Brincat, M., Hole, D., Mason, H. (2003). *Metformin has direct effects on human ovarian steroidogenesis.* Fertil Steril, ISSN 0015-0282, Elsevier, New York, USA

Mardesic, T., Muller, P., Zeťová, L., Mikova, M., Stroufová, A. (1995). *Factors affecting the results of in vitro fertilization. Importance of the stimulation protocols combining GnRH analogs and HMG in women with unsuccessful stimulation with combinations of clomiphene citrate-HMG.* Ces Gyn. ISSN 1803-6597 Praha, Czech Republic

Mitwally, M. F., Casper. (2006). *Aromatal inhibitors in ovary stimalation.* Gynek. po prom. ISSN 1213-2578 Praha, Czech Republic

Moller, DE. (1993). *Insulin resistance,* Willey, Chichester; ISBN 0471939773, Chichester New York

Moran, LJ., Strauss ,BJ., Teede, HJ. (2011). *Diabetes risk score in the diagnostic categories of polycystic ovary syndrome.* Fertil Steril. ISSN 0015-0282, Clayton, Victoria, Australia

Nader, S. (2010). *Infertility and pregnancy in women with polycystic ovary syndrome.* Minerva Endocrinologica. ISSN 0391-1977, Torino, Italy

Nasr, A. (2010). *Effect of N-acetyl-cysteine after ovarian drilling in clomiphene citrate-resistant PCOS women: a pilot study.* Reproductive Biomedicine Online, ISSN 1472-6491, New Your, NY, USA

Poppe, K., Glinoer, D. (2003). *Thyroid autoimmunity and hypothyroidism before and during pregnancy.* Hum Reprod Update, ISSN 1460-2369, Brussels, Belgium

Roberts, J., Jenkins, C., Wilson, R., et al. (1996). *Recurrent miscarriage is associated with increased numbers of CD5/20 positive lymphocytes and an increased incidence of thyroid antibodies.* Eur J Endocrinol, ISSN 0804-4643, Glasgow, UK

Roztočil, A. (2001). *Disorders of pregnancy lenght.* Porodnictví, ISBN 80-7013-339-2, Brno, Czech Republic

Schimberni, M., Morgia, F., Colabianchi, J., Giallonardo, A., Piscitelli, C., Giannini, P. (2009). *Natural-cycle in vitro fertilization in poor responder patients: a survey of 500 consecutive cycles.* Fertility & Sterility, ISSN, 0015-0282, Elsevier, New York, USA

Shahine, L.,K., Lathi, R.,B., Baker, V.,L. (2009). *Oocyte retrieval versus conversion to intrauterine insemination in patients with poor response to gonadotropin therapy.* Fertility & Sterility, ISSN: 0015-0282, Birmingham, UK

Stagnaro-Green, A., Glinoer, D. (2004). *Thyroid autoimmunity and the risk of miscarriage.* Best Pract Res Clin Endocrinol Metab, 18: 167–181. ISSN: 1521-690x, Athens, Greece

Sterzl, I., Novakova, D., Vavrejnova, V. et al. (1997) *Thyroid, ovarian and adrenal antibodies in female patients with autoimmune thyroiditis.* Cas Lek Cesk, 1997, 136(8):249, ISSN 0008-7335, Prague, Czech republic

Svačina, S. et al. (1997). *Insulin steroids and steroidogenesis.* Čs Fyziologie, ISSN: 12106313, Praha, Czech Republic

Svačina, Š. (2001). *Metabolic syndrome.* Triton, ISBN-10: 80-7254-782-8, Praha, Czech Republic

Šarapatková, H. (2008). *Actual look on polycystic ovary syndrome.* Interní Med. Pro Praxi ISSN 1212-7299 Olomouc, Czech Republic

Toscano, V. et al. (1998). *Polycystic ovary syndrome.* J of Endocr Invest, ISSN PRINT: 0391-4097, Milano, Italy

Vašičková, Z. (2003). *Obesity in gyneacology and obstetrick.* Prakt Gyn, ISSN 1801-8750, Brno, Czech Republic

Višňová, H., Ventruba, P., Crha, I. (2003). *Metformin in treatment of PCOS women.* Asist Reprod, Brno, Czech Republic

Zwinger, A. (2004). *Recurrent miscarriage.* In: Zwinger A et al. *Porodnictví.* Galén, ISBN 8072622579, Praha, Czech Republic

Žáková, J., Vetruba, P., Crha, I., Bulínová, E., Lousová, E. (2006). *Donors gamets and embryos using in infertility treatment.* Prakt Gyn, ISSN 1801-8750, Brno, Czech Republic

5

Obesity in Polycystic Ovary Syndrome

Carlos Moran[1, 3], Monica Arriaga[1],
Gustavo Rodriguez[2] and Segundo Moran[3]
[1]*Direction of Health Research and Training, Medical Unit of High Specialty, Gynecology and Obstetrics Hospital No. 4 Luis Castelazo Ayala,*
[2]*General Hospital of Zone No. 8*
[3]*Health Research Council, Mexican Institute of Social Security, Mexico City, Mexico*

1. Introduction

Polycystic ovary syndrome (PCOS) is an endocrine and metabolic heterogeneous disorder, with a likely genetic origin, influenced by environmental factors such as nutrition and physical activity. The main clinical features of PCOS are related to hyperandrogenism, such as hirsutism, acne and menstrual disorders (Moran et al., 1994; Azziz, et al., 2004; Carmina et al., 2006). PCOS is also associated with overweight or obesity (Azziz, et al., 2004), mainly abdominal adiposity (Moran et al., 1999). The etiology of PCOS is unknown. The genetic origin is based on the observation that PCOS is more frequent among the sisters and mothers of these patients (Lunde et al., 1989; Govind et al., 1999). Moreover, in a study done with twins, a higher correlation in the presence of PCOS is observed more in monozygotic than in dizygotic (Vink et al., 2006). Multiple genes related to the production of androgen, the function of the gonadotropin, the action of insulin and the regulation of energy have been evaluated. Although associations of some genes with clinical disorders of PCOS have been found, in specific regions and determined polymorphisms, the findings of studies and in different populations have not been consistent (Wood et al., 2003).

The hypothesis of the origin of PCOS by environmental factors is based on the beneficial results observed by weight loss, and the worsening with increasing weight in these patients. The interaction of environmental factors of PCOS in women affected starts from their prenatal and postnatal life (Abbott et al., 2002). Food habits and lifestyle are also factors in the presentation and the development of PCOS. The influence of the environmental component of PCOS and its interaction with the genetic component has been less studied. Obesity plays an important role in the pathogenesis of PCOS, and the majority of patients with PCOS are overweight or obese; however, these disorders are not considered as diagnostic criteria for PCOS, since not all obese women present hyperandrogenism.

2. Diagnosis

The major criteria of PCOS, proposed in the consensus of the National Institutes of Health in Bethesda, M.D., were (in order of importance): a) hyperandrogenism and/or hyperandrogenemia, b) oligoovulation, c) exclusion of other known disorders, and d) possibly the characteristic morphology of polycystic ovaries on ultrasound (Zawadzki & Dunaif, 1992). At the Rotterdam consensus, the presence of two out of the three following criteria was considered as diagnostic for PCOS: a) oligoovulation or anovulation, b) clinical and/or biochemical signs of hyperandrogenism, and c) polycystic ovaries by ultrasound, after exclusion of other related disturbances (ESHRE/ASRM-Sponsored PCOS Consensus, 2004). The Androgen Excess and PCOS Society considers as PCOS: hyperandrogenism (hirsutism and/or hyperandrogenemia), ovarian dysfunction (oligo-anovulation and/or polycystic ovaries), and the exclusion of other androgen excess or related disorders (Azziz, et al., 2006).

3. Phenotypes

Overweight and obesity are not considered for PCOS phenotypes (Azziz, et al., 2006). Phenotypes of PCOS patients can be classified as follows: A) hyperandrogenism, oligo-anovulation and polycystic ovaries by ultrasound; B) hyperandrogenism and oligo-anovulation (and normal appearance of the ovaries by ultrasound); C) hyperandrogenism and polycystic ovaries by ultrasound (with regular ovulatory menstrual cycles); and D) oligo-anovulation and polycystic ovaries by ultrasound (without hyperandrogenism). The National Institutes of Health criteria recognizes A and B phenotypes. The Rotterdam ESHRE/ASRM-Sponsored PCOS Consensus Workshop Group accepts all these phenotypes. The AE-PCOS Society admits A, B and C phenotypes (Table 1). However, each one of the phenotypes can be subdivided considering the presence of obesity, when body mass index is (BMI) ≥ 27.

Features	A1 Obese	A2 Non obese	B1 Obese	B2 Non obese	C1 Obese	C2 Non obese
Hyperandrogenism	Yes	Yes	Yes	Yes	Yes	Yes
Oligo-anovulation	Yes	Yes	Yes	Yes	No	No
Polycystic ovaries	Yes	Yes	No	No	Yes	Yes
No. %	83 48.3	28 16.3	39 22.7	17 9.9	3 1.7	2 1.2

Table 1. Phenotype classification in 172 patients with polycystic ovary syndrome taking into account obesity (body mass index ≥ 27) to subdivide each group. The frequencies of different phenotypes are unpublished data yet, Moran C, 2011.

4. Prevalence of PCOS and/or obesity

Polycystic ovary syndrome (PCOS) affects 4-7% of women in reproductive age (Knochenhauer et al., 1998; Diamanti-Kandarakis et al., 1999; Asuncion et al., 2000; Moran et al., 2010). It is considered one of the most frequent endocrine disorders in women of reproductive age (Moran et al., 2010). It is noteworthy that PCOS affects 60-80% of the patients with hyperandrogenism (Table 2) (Moran et al., 1994; Azziz et al., 2004, Carmina et al., 2006). Overweight or obesity affects approximately 60-80% of PCOS patients (Azziz et al., 2004).

Diagnosis	Mexico[1] (n = 250) %	USA[2] (n = 873) %	Italy[3] (n = 950) %
Polycystic ovary syndrome	53.6	82.0	56.6
Idiopathic hirsutism/hyperandrogenism	24.8	4.5	7.6/15.8
Overweight or obesity*	18.0	---	---
Hyperandrogenism and ovulation	---	6.7	15.5
Classic/Non classic CAH	2.0	0.7/2.1	4.3
Androgen secreting tumors	0.8	0.2	0.2
HAIRAN syndrome	---	3.8	---
Cushing's syndrome	0.4	---	---
Iatrogenic hirsutism	0.4	---	---

Table 2. Classification of hyperandrogenism in women. PCOS: polycystic ovary syndrome, CAH: Congenital adrenal hyperplasia, HAIRAN: Hyperandrogenisim, insulin resistance and acanthosis *nigricans*. *Hyperandrogenic overweight or obese patients with regular menstrual cycles. Taken from [1]Moran et al., *Archives of Medical Research*, 1994; [2]Azziz et al., *The Journal of Clinical Endocrinology & Metabolism*, 2004; [3]Carmina et al., *The Journal of Clinical Endocrinology & Metabolism*, 2006.

5. Clinical presentation in obese and nonobese PCOS patients

It has been reported that obese PCOS patients have a greater prevalence of some clinical manifestations, such as hirsutism and menstrual disorders (Kiddy et al., 1990); however, other studies have not found differences (Singh et al., 1994). The discrepancies between these studies may be the result of different diagnostic criteria used to classify obesity and PCOS.

6. Role of obesity in the pathophysiology of PCOS

6.1 Gonadotropic dysfunction

The main pathophysiological components of PCOS are gonadotropic dysfunction and insulin resistance (Dale et al., 1992; Fulghesu et al., 1999; Moran et al., 2003). It has been found that both of these components are related to BMI.

Dissociation of luteinizing hormone (LH) to follicle-stimulating hormone (FSH) higher in PCOS patients with normal weight than in obese PCOS patients has been observed in some studies (Dale et al., 1992); although this observation has not been found in other studies (Fulghesu et al., 1999; Moran et al., 2003) (Table 3).

6.2 Insulin resistance

PCOS is associated to metabolic disorders like insulin resistance (Matteini et al., 1982; Chang et al., 1983; Shoupe et al., 1983; Pasquali, et al., 1983), becoming a risk factor for development of carbohydrate intolerance and type 2 diabetes *mellitus* (Legro et al., 1999; Ehrmann et al., 1999). Insulin resistance appears in women with PCOS with suitable weight (Chang et al., 1983), and overweight or obesity (Moran et al., 2003), but is more frequent and of greater magnitude when there is obesity (Dunaif et al., 1989; Moran et al., 2003). The insulin resistance is approximately two-fold that of non obese PCOS patients (Table 3) (Moran et al., 2003). The magnitude of overweight and obesity is directly related to insulin resistance in PCOS patients (Figure 1) (Moran et al., 2003).

Disorder	PCOS with obesity %	PCOS without obesity %	Total %
Gonadotropic dysfunction LH/FSH ≥ 2	19	25	22
Insulin resistance Insulin/Glucose ≥ 28.6 (pmol/mmol)	63*	31*	47

Table 3. Frequency of pathophysiologic components of polycystic ovary syndrome (PCOS). All the determinations were performed in one sample in fasting conditions. *Statistically significant difference (P< 0.01). From Moran et al, *Fertility and Sterility*, 2003.

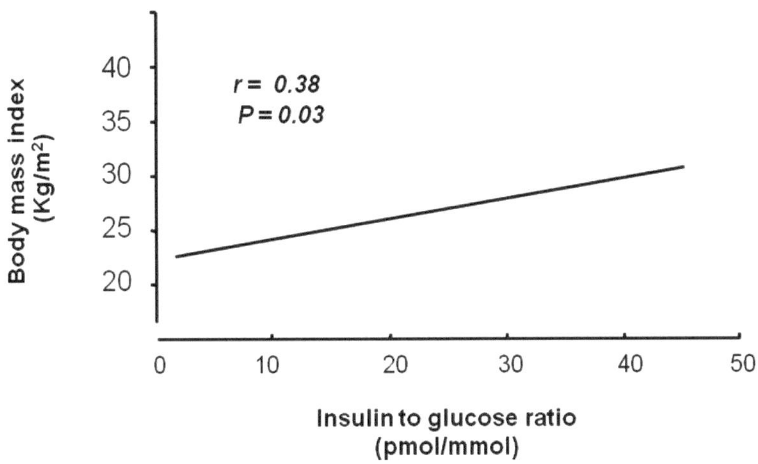

Fig. 1. Relationship between body mass and insulin resistance in patients with polycystic ovary syndrome. Modified from Moran et al, *Fertility and Sterility*, 2003.

6.3 Body fat distribution

Obesity is associated mainly to abdominal adiposity in PCOS patients (Moran et al., 2003). It is important to recognize the presence of obesity and its upper body distribution or abdominal adiposity, which changes in accordance to race and geographical distribution (ESHRE/ASRM-Sponsored PCOS Consensus, 2004). The upper body adiposity is related to insulin resistance in PCOS patients (Figure 2) (Moran et al., 2003). To this matter, upper body adiposity has been found to be associated with a higher percentage of anovulation in comparison to lower body adiposity (83% vs. 65%, respectively) (Moran et al., 1999).

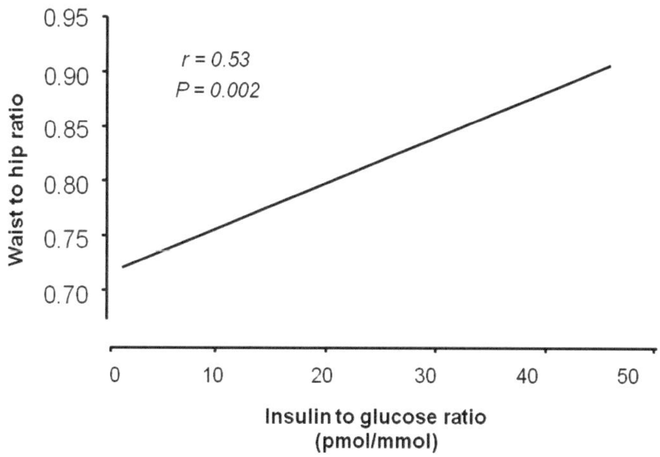

Fig. 2. Relationship between body fat distribution and insulin resistance in patients with polycystic ovary syndrome. Modified from Moran et al, *Fertility and Sterility*, 2003.

6.4 Ovarian morphology of polycystic ovaries

There is some evidence indicating the relationship of anthropometric and hormonal measures with the characteristic polycystic ovarian morphology. On analyzing the anthropometric variables of PCOS patients, BMI is significantly greater in PCOS patients with a characteristic polycystic ovary image than in those without it; also, it has been found that the hip perimeter is significantly greater in PCOS patients with characteristic image of polycystic ovary than in those without this ultrasonographic morphology (Tena et al., 2011). In addition, PCOS patients with the polycystic ovarian morphology by ultrasound present greater levels of testosterone than patients without it.

6.5 Adipocytokines

Patients with PCOS-in comparison to control women-present lower serum levels of adiponectin but not of leptin. A decrease was observed in the expression of the ribonucleic acid (RNA) messenger of adiponectin in the subcutaneous and visceral adipose tissue, while that of leptin has been found significantly less only in the subcutaneous adipose tissue. Also, it has been observed an inverse relationship among adiponectin and leptin expression and the measurement of subcutaneous and visceral adipose tissue by ultrasound (Carmina et al., 2008). Other authors have reported that obese PCOS but not normal weight PCOS patients have significantly lower adiponectin levels than control women (Olszanecka-Glinianowicz et al., 2011).

6.6 Metabolic syndrome

The prevalence of metabolic syndrome is higher in PCOS patients than in control women (47% vs. 4%, respectively) (Dokras et al., 2005). Free fatty acids, total cholesterol and low density lipoprotein cholesterol are higher in obese PCOS patients than in non obese PCOS patients (Holte et al., 1994). Both PCOS and obesity are associated with dyslipidemia and endothelial dysfunction that increase the cardiovascular risk. Although metabolic disorders prevail in the climacteric period, the risk of metabolic syndrome is high even at reproductive age.

Both PCOS and obesity induce an increase in serum inflammatory cardiovascular risk markers (Samy et al., 2009). Increased C-reactive protein, interleukin-6 and tumor necrosis factor alpha have been reported in obese PCOS patients with respect to control women; in addition, these markers have correlated with BMI and insulin resistance (Samy et al., 2009). Fatty liver has been reported present until 40% of PCOS patients associated to higher BMI, abdominal obesity and worse lipid profile (Ma et al., 2011). The pathogenetic relation among PCOS, obesity, metabolic and cardiovascular disease is controversial. A low-grade chronic inflammation has been proposed as the potential cause of the long-term complications of PCOS (Repaci et al., 2011).

7. Androgen production in obese and non obese PCOS patients

In normal women, androstenedione and testosterone are produced mainly in the ovaries, while dehydroepiandrosterone and dehydroepiandrosterone sulfate are secreted predominantly in the adrenals (Parker, 2006). The ovaries produce approximately 50% of testosterone and androstenedione while the adrenals 70% of dehydroepiandrosterone and almost all dehydroepiandrosterone sulfate (Longcope, 1986). Dehydroepiandrosterone is the main precursor of androgens and estrogens, and it is sulfated by the enzyme SULT2A1 in adrenals (Miller et al., 2006).

Controversy exists about the effect of obesity on serum androgen concentrations in PCOS. Some investigators have reported that testosterone and androstenedione levels are similar in obese and non obese PCOS patients (Dale et al., 1992; Dos Reis et al., 1995). However, it is well known that obesity generates a decrease in the sexual hormone-binding globulin (SHBG), and therefore an increase in the free androgens (Kiddy et al., 1990; Holte et al., 1994). Other studies have found that obesity generates an increase of testosterone levels in PCOS patients (Figure 3) (Holte et al., 1994; Acien et al., 1999, Moran et al., 2008). In contrast, dynamic studies have shown a decrease in androstenedione levels in obese PCOS patients (Dunaif et al., 1988; Moran et al., 2008).

Hyperandrogenism may be of ovarian or adrenal origin (Rosenfield et al., 1972). Participation in PCOS by the increment of dehydroepiandrosterone sulfate is found in 22-25% of PCOS patients (Moran et al., 1999). However, some studies have found frequencies of hyperandrogenism due to dehydroepiandrosterone sulfate of 48-52% in different populations (Carmina et al., 1992). Hyperandrogenic patients with higher adrenal androgen excess have been informed to be leaner, younger and present more hirsutism than patients with lower levels of these steroids (Moran et al., 1999).

8. Obesity in pregnant PCOS patients

Due to obesity and PCOS determine independently a deleterious effect on pregnancy and reproductive outcome, their impact of both conditions together are expectedly adverse in pregnant women and their fetuses. Obese patients with PCOS are characterized by a more severe hyperandrogenic and metabolic state, more irregular menses, less ovulatory cycles and lower pregnancy rates, compared with normal weight PCOS patients; the importance of obesity in the pathogenesis of PCOS is evidenced by the efficacy of weight loss to improve metabolic alterations, to decrease hyperandrogenism, to increase ovulatory menstrual cycles and to improve fertility (Pasquali et al., 2006). The information with respect to the impact of obesity in hormonal and metabolic factors during intrauterine life is scarce yet.

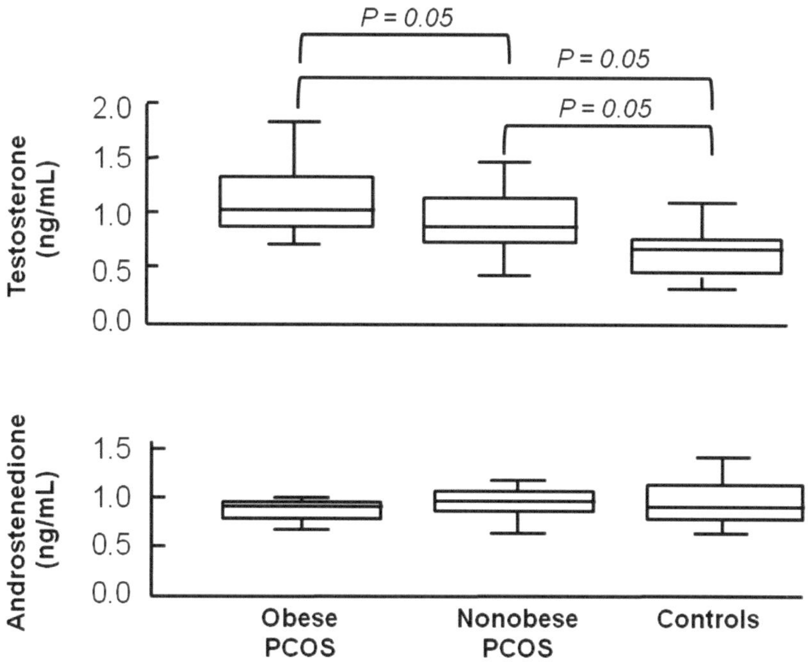

Fig. 3. Values of total testosterone and androstenedione in obese and nonobese patients with PCOS and in control women. Box-and-whiskers plots of basal levels of androgens. The line within each box represents the median. Upper and lower boundaries of each box indicate 75th and 25th percentiles, respectively. The whiskers (above and below) show the upper and lower adjacent values, respectively. The levels of testosterone were significantly greater in the obese patients with PCOS compared with non obese PCOS patients and controls. Also, the testosterone levels were significantly greater in non obese PCOS patients than in control women. There were no significant differences in the levels of androstenedione. Modified from Moran et al, *Fertility and Sterility*, 2008.

9. Treatment of obesity and metabolic abnormalities in PCOS patients

The current management of PCOS has to attend to the clinical, hormonal and metabolic abnormalities. The change in PCOS concept of the treatment is that it is not considered only a reproductive problem but also an endocrine and metabolic disorder that requires a long term follow-up. Furthermore, the treatment must address specific problems that affect PCOS patients, such as hirsutism, acne, overweight or obesity, menstrual disorders and infertility (Moran et al., 1994; Azziz et al., 2004, Carmina et al., 2006).

9.1 Modifications in life style

Weight loss is the principal recommendation as the first line of treatment in obese women with PCOS. The treatment of obesity in PCOS must include nutritional counselling in food habits and lifestyle (Kiddy et al., 1992; L.J. Moran et al., 2003). The weight loss partially ameliorates hirsutism (Pasquali et al., 1989; Kiddy et al., 1992), regularizes menstrual cycles and ovulation, as well as improves the endocrine and metabolic abnormalities (Pasquali et al., 1989; Kiddy et al., 1992; Guzick et al., 1994; Holte et al., 1995).

9.1.1 Food habit

There is a known beneficial effect of the decrease of body weight and a worsening with the increase of excess weight in PCOS patients. It has been observed that some patients with PCOS can present menstrual cycles and ovulation after having reduced at least 5 % of her body weight (Kiddy et al., 1992). The studies on food habits in patients with PCOS have shown that the most important thing is caloric restriction, achieving a reduction of about 7% body weight, and that there is no difference in the metabolic results changing the composition of the diet (L.J. Moran et al., 2003). However, it has been reported that low glycemic index diet improved insulin sensitivity and menstrual periodicity more than the conventional healthy diet in PCOS patients (Marsh, 2010).

9.1.2 Exercise

Physical activity has been shown lower in PCOS patients than in control women (Write et al., 2004). The changes in lifestyle that incorporate an increase of physical activity and limited caloric intake have been beneficial in some studies. Regular physical activity is an important component to support the reduction of long-term weight; the results are minimal with exercise alone (Hoeger, 2008). An increase in physical activity is recommended for women with obesity and PCOS, as long as cardiovascular and orthopaedic limitations are considered (Moran et al., 2006).

9.2 Insulin sensitizer agents

9.2.1 Metformin

The temporary use of metformin is considered, as a coadjutant of diet and exercise to control insulin resistance, especially in patients with obesity and glucose intolerance (Velazquez et al., 1994; ESHRE/ASRM-Sponsored PCOS Consensus Workshop Group, 2008). Nevertheless, the duration of this therapy is unknown yet. The metformin diminishes the hepatic glucose synthesis, inhibiting the gluconeogenesis; it also increases the glucose use by the striated muscle (Kirpichnikow et al., 2002).

Administration of metformin to obese PCOS patients reduces the levels of circulating insulin, the activity of the complex P450c17α and the ovarian secretion of androgens (Nestler & Jakubowicz, 1996). Metformin can reduce the circulating androgen levels, may normalize the menstrual cycles and improve ovulation (Velazquez et al., 1994). The combined use of metformin and clomiphene has been recommended for PCOS patients with overweight or obesity who present more insulin resistance, especially in those refractory to the clomiphene (ESHRE/ASRM-Sponsored PCOS Consensus Workshop Group, 2008).

Metformin has contraindications and some side effects (Lord et al., 2003). It must not be used in patients with renal insufficiency, hepatic malfunction, congestive heart failure and those with a history of alcoholism. It is important to take into account that metformin in rare cases can produce lactic acidosis; it is necessary to evaluate renal function before and periodically during its administration, even though this complication is extremely rare. The gastrointestinal adverse effects, mainly nausea and diarrhoea, affect 10 to 25% of the patients taking metformin. The undesirable effects are transitory; however, in a minority of patients these can cause discontinuation of the treatment. To minimize adverse effects, metformin must be administered gradually. Metformin can induce bad absorption of vitamin B12 in patients who use it for long periods of time, even though this effect is very rare. In patients who wish to use contraception, it is necessary to add an oral contraceptive while still taking metformin. In those cases of hirsutism it is possible to add antiandrogens, oral contraceptives or both.

9.2.2 Thiazolidindiones

Among thiazolidindiones are troglitazone, rosiglitazone and pioglitazone, which improve the sensitivity of the insulin in the liver, striated muscle and adipose tissue; they also reduce the concentrations of insulin and circulating androgens (Lord et al., 2003). The use of troglitazone was ceased in research protocols conducted in PCOS patients because of hepatotoxicity reports. Although rosiglitazone and pioglitazone are as effective as metformin to treat insulin resistance in PCOS patients, it appears they are less effective to lower BMI than metformin. These drugs have been used less due to the concern of their use during pregnancy.

9.3 Drugs for obesity and dyslipidemia

Drugs to control obesity have been used in obese patients with PCOS, although few studies exist to support this therapeutic approach. It is known that orlistat blocks the absorption of intestinal fat (Jayagopa et al., 2005), and sibutramine suppresses the appetite (Sabunku et al., 2003); both favor weight loss independently from the androgen excess and insulin resistance. It is important to take into account that these treatments must not be considered first line treatments for obesity in patients with PCOS.

There are little evidences that statins, apart from specific action on lipid profile decreasing total cholesterol and low density lipoprotein cholesterol, can reduce serum androgens, inflammatory markers and insulin resistance (Banaszewska et al., 2009; Sathyapalan et al., 2009, Raja-Khan et al., 2011). However, statins and bezafibrate (Hara et al., 2010) should only be used in women with PCOS who meet current indications for those treatments.

9.4 Bariatric surgery

Few studies exist on the impact of bariatric weight loss surgery on manifestations of PCOS in patients with morbid obesity. The initial results of bariatric surgery in patients with morbid obesity and PCOS seem encouraging, since aside from the weight reduction there is a decrease of hyperandrogenemia, hirsutism, insulin resistance and restoration of menstrual cycles and ovulation (Escobar-Morreale et al., 2005).

10. Research of obesity and PCOS for the future

The differences in the hormonal and metabolic profile, as well as the different response to treatment of obese and non obese PCOS patients suggest that obesity has to be considered as a secondary characteristic for the PCOS phenotype classification in prospective trials.

The intrauterine milieu in pregnancy and the reproduction outcome of PCOS patients with overweight or obesity are important topics for research in prospective studies.

PCOS and obesity induce an increase in serum inflammatory cardiovascular risk markers. The precise mechanisms underlying these associations require additional studies, to determine the relative contribution of different factors on cardiovascular disease.

11. Summary

PCOS is associated with overweight or obesity, mainly abdominal adiposity; approximately 80% of patients with PCOS are either overweight or obese. The insulin resistance, present in most of patients with obesity and/or PCOS, is a risk factor to develop carbohydrate intolerance and type 2 diabetes *mellitus*. Insulin resistance is higher and of greater magnitude in obese than non obese PCOS patients. A decrease in the synthesis of SHBG has been found, and therefore an increase in the free androgens in obese PCOS patients. It has been observed in some studies that obese PCOS patients present an increase of testosterone levels and a decrease in androstenedione. Weight loss is the main recommendation in obese PCOS patients. The treatment of obesity in PCOS must include nutritional counselling in food habits and life style. An increase in physical activity is recommended for PCOS patients. The temporary use of metformin may be useful, in conjunction with diet and exercise, to control insulin resistance, especially in PCOS patients with obesity and glucose intolerance. The combined use of metformin and clomiphene for ovulation induction has been suggested mainly in patients with overweight or obesity, who present more insulin resistance, refractory to the clomiphene alone. Drugs used to control obesity, as orlistat or sibutramine, must not be considered as the first choice for obesity in patients with PCOS. The initial results of bariatric surgery in patients with morbid obesity and PCOS seem encouraging, since aside from the weight reduction, a decrease of hyperandrogenemia, insulin resistance, hirsutism, and the restoration of menstrual cycles and ovulation have been observed. Obesity decreases or delays the results of several treatments for infertility such as the administration of clomiphene, gonadotropins and ovarian drilling. The differences in the hormonal and metabolic profile, as well as the different response to treatment between obese and non obese PCOS patients suggest that obesity has to be considered as a secondary characteristic for the determination of PCOS phenotypes.

12. Acknowledgments

The authors would like to thank Jaime Rodríguez, Manuel Mendez, Aida Moran, Maria Basavilvazo and Jennifer Pannebecker, for their kind technical help in the edition of this manuscript.

13. References

Abbott, D.H.; Dumesic, D.A. & Franks, S. (2002). Developmental origin of polycystic ovary syndrome - a hypothesis. *Journal of Endocrinology*, Vo.l. 174, No. 1, pp. 1-5, ISSN 0022-0795

Acien, P.; Quereda, F.; Matallin, P.; Villarroya, E.; Lopez-Fernandez, J.A.; Acien, M.; Mauri, M. & Alfayate R. (1999). Insulin, androgens, and obesity in women with and without polycystic ovary syndrome: a heterogeneous group of disorders. *Fertility and Sterility*, Vol. 72, No. 1, pp. 32-40, ISSN 0015-0282

Asuncion, M.; Calvo, R.M.; San Millan, J.L.; Sancho, J.; Avila, S. & Escobar-Morreale, H.F. (2000). A prospective study of the prevalence of the polycystic ovary syndrome in unselected caucasian women from Spain. *The Journal of Clinical Endocrinology & Metabolism*, Vol. 85, No. 7, pp. 2434-2438, ISSN 0021-972X

Azziz, R.; Carmina, E.; Dewailly, D.; Diamanti-Kandarakis, E.; Escobar-Morreale, H.F.; Futterweit, W.; Janssen, O.E.; Legro, R.S.; Norman, R.J.; Taylor, A.E. & Witchel, S.F. (2006). Position statement: criteria for defining polycystic ovary syndrome as a predominantly hyperandrogenic syndrome: an Androgen Excess Society Guideline. *The Journal of Clinical Endocrinology & Metabolism*, Vol. 91, No. 11, pp. 4237-4245, ISSN 0021-972X

Azziz, R.; Sanchez, L.A.; Knochenhauer, E.S.; Moran, C.; Lazenby, J.; Stephens, K.C.; Taylor, K. & Boots, L.R. (2004). Androgen excess in women: experience with over 1000 consecutive patients. *The Journal of Clinical Endocrinology & Metabolism*, Vol. 89, No. 2, pp. 453-462, ISSN 0021-972X

Banaszewska, B.; Pawelczyk, L.; Spaczynski, R.Z. & Duleba, A. J. (2009). Comparison of simvastatin and metformin in treatment of polycystic ovary syndrome: prospective randomized trial. *The Journal of Clinical Endocrinology & Metabolism*, Vol. 94, No. 12, pp. 4938-4945, ISSN 0021-972X

Carmina, E.; Koyama, T.; Chang, L.; Stanczyk, F.Z. & Lobo, R.A. (1992). Does ethnicity influence the prevalence of adrenal hyperandrogenism and insulin resistance in polycystic ovary syndrome? *American Journal of Obstetrics and Gynecology*, Vol. 167, No. 6, pp. 1807-1812, ISSN 0002-9378

Carmina, E.; Chu, M.C.; Moran, C.; Tortoriello, D.; Vardhana, P.; Tena, G.; Preciado, R. & Lobo, R. (2008). Subcutaneous and omental fat expression of adiponectin and leptin in women with polycystic ovary syndrome. *Fertility and Sterility*, Vol. 89, No. 3, pp. 642-648, ISSN 0015-0282

Carmina, E.; Rosato, F.; Janni, A.; Rizzo, M. & Longo, R.A. (2006). Relative prevalence of different androgen excess disorders in 950 women referred because of clinical hyperandrogenism. *The Journal of Clinical Endocrinology & Metabolism*, Vol. 91, No. 1, pp. 2-6, ISSN 0021-972X

Chang, R.J.; Nakamura, R.M.; Judd, H.L. & Kaplan, S.A. (1983). Insulin resistance in nonobese patients with polycystic ovarian disease. *The Journal of Clinical Endocrinology & Metabolism*, Vol. 57, No. 2, pp. 356-359, ISSN 0021-972X

Dale, P.O.; Tanbo, T.; Vaaler, S. & Abyholm, T. (1992). Body weight, hyperinsulinemia, and gonadotropin levels in the polycystic ovarian syndrome: evidence of two distinct populations. *Fertility and Sterility*, Vol. 58, No. 3, pp. 487-491, ISSN 0015-0282

Diamanti-Kandarakis, E.; Kouli, C.R.; Bergiele, A.T.; Filandra, F.A.; Tsianateli, T.C.; Spina, G.G.; Zapanti, E.D. & Bartzis, M.I. (1999). A survey of the polycystic ovary syndrome in the Greek Island of Lesbos: hormonal and metabolic profile. *The Journal of Clinical Endocrinology & Metabolism*, Vol. 84, No. 11, pp. 4006-4011, ISSN 0021-972X

Dokras, A.; Bochner, M; Hollinrake, E.; Markham, S.; Vanvoorhis, B. & Jagasia, D.H. (2005). Screening women with polycystic ovary syndrome for metabolic syndrome. *Obstetrics and Gynecology*, Vol. 106, No. 1, pp.131-137, ISSN 0029-7844

Dos Reis, R.M.; Foss, M.C.; Dias de Moura, M.; Ferriani, R.A. & Silva de Sa, M.F. (1995). Insulin secretion in obese and non-obese women with polycystic ovary syndrome and its relationship with hyperandrogenism. *Gynecological Endocrinology*, Vol. 9, No. 1, pp. 45-50, ISSN 0951-3590

Dunaif, A.; Mandeli, J.; Fluhr, H. & Dobrjansky, A. (1988). The impact of obesity and chronic hyperinsulinemia on gonadotropin realease and gonadal steroid secretion in the polycystic ovary syndrome. *The Journal of Clinical Endocrinology & Metabolism*, Vol. 66, No. 1, pp. 131-139, ISSN 0021-972X

Dunaif, A.; Segal, K.R.; Futterweit, W. & Dobrjansky, A. (1989). Profound peripheral insulin resistance, independent of obesity, in polycystic ovary syndrome. *Diabetes*, Vol. 38, No. 9, pp. 1165-1174, ISSN 0012-1797

Ehrmann, D.A.; Barnes, R.B.; Rosenfield, R.L.; Cavaghan, M.K. & Imperial, J. (1999). Prevalence of impaired glucose tolerance and diabetes in women with polycystic ovary syndrome. *Diabetes Care*, Vol. 22, No. 1, pp. 141-146, ISSN 0149-5992

Escobar- Morreale, H.F.; Botella-Carretero, J.I.; Alvarez-Blasco, F.; Sancho, J. & San Millan, J.L. (2005). The polycystic ovary syndrome associated with morbid obesity may resolve after weight loss induced by bariatric surgery. *The Journal of Clinical Endocrinology & Metabolism*, Vol. 90, No. 12, pp. 6364-6369, ISSN 0021-972X

Fulghesu, A.M.; Cucinelli, F.; Pavone, V.; Murgia, F.; Guido, M.; Caruso, A.; Mancuso, S. & Lanzone, A. (1999). Changes in luteinizing hormone and insulin secretion in polycystic ovarian syndrome. *Human Reproduction*, Vol. 14, No. 3, pp. 611-617, ISSN 0268-1161

Govind, A.; Obhrai, M.S. & Clayton, R.N. (1999). Polycystic ovaries are inherited as an autosomal dominant trait: analysis of 29 polycystic ovary syndrome and 10 control families. *The Journal of Clinical Endocrinology & Metabolism*, Vol. 84, No. 1, pp. 38-43, ISSN 0021-972X

Guzick, D.S.; Wing, R.; Smith, D.; Berga, S.L. & Winters, S.J. (1994). Endocrine consequences of weight loss in obese, hyperandrogenic, anovulatory women. *Fertility and Sterility*, Vol. 61, No. 4, pp. 598-604, ISSN 0015-0282

Hara, S.; Takahashi, T.; Amita, M.; Igarashi, S. & Kurachi H. (2010). Usefulness of bezafibrate for ovulation induction in clomiphene citrate-resistant polycystic ovary syndrome patients with dyslipidemia: a prospective pilot study of seven cases. *Gynecologic and Obstetric Investigation*, Vol. 70, No. 3, pp. 166-172, ISSN 0378-7346

Hoeger, K.M. (2008). Exercise therapy in polycystic ovary syndrome. *Seminars in Reproductive Medicine* Vol. 26, No. 1, pp. 93-100, ISSN 1526-8004

Holte, J.; Bergh, T.; Berne, C. & Lithell, H. (1994). Serum lipoprotein lipid profile in women with the polycystic ovary syndrome: relation to anthropometric, endocrine and metabolic variables. *Clinical Endocrinology*, Vol. 41, No. 4, pp 463-471, ISSN 0300-0664

Holte, J.; Bergh, T.; Berne, C.; Wide, L. & Lithell, H. (1995). Restored insulin sensitivity but persistently increased early insulin secretion after weight loss in obese women with polycystic ovary syndrome. *The Journal of Clinical Endocrinology & Metabolism*, Vol. 80, No. 9, pp. 2586-2593, ISSN 0021-972X

Jayagopal, V.; Kilpatrick, E.S.; Holding, S.; Jennings, P.E. & Atkin,S.L. (2005). Orlistat is as beneficial as metformin in the treatment of polycystic ovarian syndrome. *The Journal of Clinical Endocrinology & Metabolism*, Vol. 90, No. 2, pp. 729-733, ISSN 0021-972X

Kiddy, D.S.; Hamilton-Fairley, D.; Bush, A.; Short, F.; Anyaoku, V.; Reed, M.J. & Franks, S. (1992). Improvement in endocrine and ovarian function during dietary treatment of obese women with polycystic ovary syndrome. *Clinical Endocrinology* Vol. 36, No. 1, pp. 105-111, ISSN 0300-0664

Kiddy, D.S.; Sharp, P.S.; White, D.M.; Scanlon, M.F.; Mason, H.D.; Bray, C.S.; Polson, D.W.; Reed, M.J. & Franks, S. (1990). Differences in clinical and endocrine features between obese and non-obese subjects with polycystic ovary syndrome: an analysis of 263 consecutive cases. *Clinical Endocrinology,* Vol. 32, No. 2, pp. 213-220, ISSN 0300-0664

Kirpichnikov, D.; McFarlane, S.I. & Sowers, J.R. (2002). Metformin: an update. *Annals of Internal Medicine,* Vol. 137, No. 1, pp. 25-33, ISSN 0003-4819

Knochenhauer, E.S.; Key, T.J.; Kahsar-Miller, M.; Waggoner, W.; Boots, L.R. & Azziz, R. (1998). Prevalence of the polycystic ovary syndrome in unselected Black and White women of the southeastern United States: a prospective study. *The Journal of Clinical Endocrinology & Metabolism,* Vol. 83, No. 9, pp. 3078-3082, ISSN 0021-972X

Legro, R.S.; Kunselman, A.R.; Dodson, W.C. & Dunaif, A. (1999). Prevalence and predictors of risk for type 2 diabetes mellitus and impaired glucose tolerance in polycystic ovary syndrome: a prospective, controlled study in 254 affected women. *The Journal of Clinical Endocrinology & Metabolism,* Vol. 84, No. 1, pp.165-169, ISSN 0021-972X

Longcope, C. (1986). Adrenal and gonadal androgen secretion in normal females. *The Journal of Clinical Endocrinology & Metabolism,* Vol. 15, No. 2, pp. 213-228, ISSN 0021-972X

Lord, J.M.; Flight, I.H. & Norman, R.J. (2003). Insulin-sensitising drugs (metformin, troglitazone, rosiglitazone, pioglitazone, D-chiro-inositol) for polycystic ovary syndrome. *Cochrane Database System Review,* 3:CD003053, ISSN 1469-493X

Lunde, O.; Magnus, P.; Sandvik, L. & Hoglo, S. (1989). Familial clustering in the polycystic ovary syndrome. *Gynecologic and Obstetric Investigation,* Vol. 28, No. 1, pp.23-30, ISSN 0378-7346

Ma, R.C.; Liu, K.H.; Lam, P.M.; Cheung, L.P.; Tam, W.H.; Ko, G.T.; Chan, M.H.; Ho, C.S.; Lam, C.W.; Chu, W.C.; Tong, P.C.; So, W.Y.; Chan, J.C. & Chow C.C. (2011). Sonographic measurement of mesenteric fat predicts presence of fatty liver among subjects with polycystic ovary syndrome. *The Journal of Clinical Endocrinology & Metabolism,* Vol. 96, No. 3, pp.799-807, ISSN 0021-972X

Marsh, K.A.; Steinbeck, K.S.; Atkinson, F.S.; Petocz, P. & Brand-Miller, J.C. (2010). Effect of a low glycemic index compared with a conventional healthy diet on polycystic ovary syndrome. *American Journal of Clinical Nutrition,* Vol. 92, No. 1, pp. 83-92, ISSN: 0002-9165

Matteini, M.; Cortrozzi, G.; Bufalini G.N.; Relli, P. & Lazzari, T. (1982). Hyperinsulinism and insulin resistance in the polycystic ovary syndrome as tested with tolbutamide. *Bollettino Societa Italiana Biologia Sperimentale,* Vol. 58, No. 22, pp. 1455-1460 ISNN 0037-8771

Miller, W.L.; Geller, D.H. & Rosen, M. (2006). Ovarian and adrenal androgen biosynthesis and metabolism. In: *Androgen excess disorders in women. Polycystic ovary syndrome and other disorders,* R. Azziz, J.E. Nestler & D. Dewailly (Eds.). Second edition. Human Press, ISBN 1-59745-179-7, Totowa, NJ, USA. Ch.2, pp. 19-33

Moran, C.; Garcia-Hernandez, E.; Barahona, E.; Gonzalez, S. & Bermudez, J.A. (2003). Relationship between insulin resistance and gonadotropin dissociation in obese and nonobese women with polycystic ovary syndrome. *Fertility and Sterility*, Vol. 80, No. 6, pp. 1466-1472, ISSN 0015-0282

Moran, C.; Hernandez, E.; Ruiz, J.E.; Fonseca, M.E.; Bermudez, J.A. & Zarate, A. (1999). Upper body obesity and hyperinsulinemia are associated with anovulation. *Gynecologic and Obstetric Investigation*, Vol. 47, No. 1, pp.1-5, ISSN 0378-7346

Moran, C.; Knochenhauer, E.S.; Boots, L.R. & Azziz, R. (1999). Adrenal androgen excess in hyperandrogenism: relation to age and body mass. *Fertility and Sterility*, Vol. 71, No. 4, pp. 671-674, ISSN 0015-0282

Moran, C.; Renteria, J.L.; Moran, S.; Herrera, J.; Gonzalez, S. & Bermudez, J.A. (2008). Obesity differentially affects serum levels of androstenedione and testosterone in polycystic ovary syndrome. *Fertility and Sterility*, Vol. 90, No. 6, pp. 2310-2317, ISSN 0015-0282

Moran, C.; Tapia, M.C.; Hernandez, E.; Vazquez, G.; Garcia Hernandez, E. & Bermudez, J.A. (1994). Etiological review of hirsutism in 250 patients. *Archives of Medical Research*, Vol. 25, No. 3, pp. 311-314, ISSN 0188-4409

Moran, C.; Tena, G.; Moran, S.; Ruiz, P.; Reyna, R. & Duque X. (2010). Prevalence of polycystic ovary syndrome and related disorders in Mexican women. *Gynecologic and Obstetric Investigation*, Vol. 69, No. 4, pp. 274-280, ISSN 0378-7346

Moran, L.J.; Brinkworth, G.; Noakes, M. & Norman, R.J. (2006). Effects of lifestyle modification in polycystic ovarian syndrome. *Reproductive Biomedicine Online*, Vol. 12, No. 5, pp. 569-578, ISNN 1472-6483

Moran, L.J.; Noakes, M.; Clifton, P.M.; Tomlinson, L.; Galletly, C. & Norman, R.J. (2003). Dietary composition in restoring reproductive and metabolic physiology in overweight women with polycystic ovary syndrome. *The Journal of Clinical Endocrinology & Metabolism*, Vol. 88, No. 2, pp. 812-819, ISSN 0021-972X

Nestler, J.E. & Jakubowicz, D.J. (1996). Decreases in ovarian cytochrome P450c17α activity and serum free testosterone after reduction of insulin secretion in polycystic ovary syndrome. *New England Journal of Medicine*, Vol. 335, No. 9, pp. 617-623, ISSN 0028-4793

Olszanecka-Glinianowicz, M.; Kuglin, D.; Dabkowska-Huc, A & Skalba P. (2011). Serum adiponectin and resistin in relation to insulin resistance and markers of hyperandrogenism in lean and obese women with polycystic ovary syndrome. *European Journal of Obstetrics & Gynecology and Reproductive Biology*, Vol. 154, No. 1, pp. 51-56, ISSN 0301-2115

Parker, Jr. C.R. (2006). Androgens throughout the life of women. In: *Androgen excess disorders in women. Polycystic ovary syndrome and other disorders*, R. Azziz, J.E. Nestler, & D. Dewailly (Eds.). Second edition. Human Press, ISBN 1-59745-179-7, Totowa, NJ, USA. Ch.3, pp. 35-47

Pasquali, R.; Antenucci, D.; Casimirri, F.; Venturoli, S.; Paradisi, F.; Fabbri, R.; Balestra, B.; Melchionda N.; & Barbara L. (1989). Clinical and hormonal characteristics of obese amenorrheic hyperandrogenic women before and after weight loss. *The Journal of Clinical Endocrinology & Metabolism*, Vol. 68, No. 1, pp. 173-179, ISSN 0021-972X

Pasquali, R.; Casimirri, F.; Venturoli, S.; Paradisi, R.; Mattioli, L.; Capelli, M.; Melchionda, N. & Labo, G. (1983). Insulin resistance in patients with polycystic ovaries: its relationship to body weight and androgen levels. *Acta Endocrinologica*, Vol. 104, No. 1, pp. 110-116, ISSN 0001-5598

Pasquali, R.; Gambineri, A. & Pagotto, U. (2006). The impact of obesity on reproduction in women with polycystic ovary syndrome. *British Journal of Obstetrics and Gynaecology*, Vol. 113, No. 10, pp. 148-159, ISSN 1471-0528

Raja-Khan, N.; Kunselman, A.R.; Hogeman, C.S.; Stetter, C.M.; Demers L.M. & Legro R.S. (2011). Effects of atorvastatin on vascular function, inflammation, and androgens in women with polycystic ovary syndrome: a double-blind, randomized, placebo-controlled trial. *Fertility and Sterility*, Vol. 95, No. 5, pp.1849-1852, ISSN 0015-0282

Repaci, A.; Gambineri, A. & Pasquali, R. (2011). The role of low-grade inflammation in the polycystic ovary syndrome. *Molecular and Cellular Endocrinology*, Vol. 335, No. 1, pp. 30-41, ISSN 0303-7207

Rosenfield, R.L.; Ehrlich, E.N. & Cleary, R.E. (1972). Adrenal and ovarian contributions to the elevated free plasma androgen levels in hirsute women. *The Journal of Clinical Endocrinology & Metabolism*, Vol. 34, No. 1, pp. 92-98, ISSN 0021-972X

Sabuncu, T.; Harma, M.; Harma, M.; Nazligul, Y. & Kilic, F. (2003). Sibutramine has a positive effect on clinical and metabolic parameters in obese patients with polycystic ovary syndrome. *Fertility and Sterility*, Vol. 80, No. 5, pp.1199-1204, ISSN 0015-0282

Samy, M.; Hashim, M.; Sayed, M. & Said, M. (2009). Clinical significance of inflammatory markers in polycystic ovary syndrome; their relationship to insulin resistance and body mass index. *Disease Markers*, Vol. 26, No. 4, pp.163-170, ISSN 0278-0240

Sathyapalan, T.; Kilpatrick, E.S.; Coady, A.M. & Atkin, S.L. (2009). The effect of atorvastatin in patients with polycystic ovary syndrome: a randomized double-blind placebo-controlled study. *The Journal of Clinical Endocrinology & Metabolism*, Vol. 94, No. 1, pp. 103-108, ISSN 0021-972X

Shoupe, D.; Kumar, D.D. & Lobo, R.A. (1983). Insulin resistance in polycystic ovary syndrome. *American Journal of Obstetrics and Gynecology*, Vol. 147, No. 5, pp. 588-592, ISSN 0002-9378

Singh, K.B.; Mahajan, D.K. & Wortsman, J. (1994). Effect of obesity on the clinical and hormonal characteristics of the polycystic ovary syndrome. *Journal of Reproductive Medicine*, Vol. 39, No. 10, pp. 805-808, ISSN 0024-7758

Tena, G.; Moran, C.; Romero, R. & Moran, S. (2011). Ovarian morphology and endocrine function in polycystic ovary syndrome. *Archives of Gynecology and Obstetrics* Vol. 284, No. 6, pp. 1443-1448, ISSN 0932-0067

The Rotterdam ESHRE/ASRM-Sponsored PCOS Consensus Workshop Group. (2004). Revised 2003 consensus on diagnostic criteria and long-term health risks related to polycystic ovary syndrome. *Fertility and Sterility*, Vol. 81, No. 1, pp. 19-24, ISSN 0015-0282

The Thessaloniki ESHRE/ASRM-Sponsored PCOS Consensus Workshop Group. (2008). Consensus on infertility treatment related to polycystic ovary syndrome. *Fertility and Sterility*, Vol. 89, No. 3, pp.: 505-522, ISSN 0015-0282

Velazquez, E.M.; Mendoza, S.; Hamer, T.; Sosa, F. & Glueck, C.J. (1994). Metformin therapy in polycystic ovary syndrome reduces hyperinsulinemia, insulin resistance, hyperandrogenemia, and systolic blood pressure, while facilitating normal menses and preganancy. *Metabolism*, Vol. 43, No. 5, pp. 647-654, ISSN 0026-0495

Vink, J.M.; Sadrzadeh, S.; Lambalk, C.B. & Boomsma, D.I. (2006). Heritability of polycystic ovary syndrome in a Dutch twin-family study. *The Journal of Clinical Endocrinology & Metabolism*, Vol. 91, No. 6, pp. 2100-2104, ISSN 0021-972X

Wright, C.E.; Zborowski, J.V.; Talbott, E.O.; McHugh-Pemu, K. & Youk, A. (2004). Dietary intake, physical activity and obesity in women with polycystic ovary syndrome. *International Journal of Obesity and Related Metabolic Disorders*, Vol. 28, No. 8, pp.1026-1032, ISNN 0307-0565

Wood, J.R.; Nelson, V.L.; Ho, C.; Jansen, E.; Wang, C.Y.; Urbanek, M.; McAllister, J.M.; Mosselman, S. & Srauss III, J.F. (2003). The molecular phenotype of polycystic ovary syndrome (PCOS) theca cells and new candidate PCOS genes defined by microarray analysis. *Journal of Biological Chemistry*, Vol. 278, No. 29, pp. 26380-26390, ISSN 0021-9258

Zawadzki, J.K. & Dunaif, A. (1992). Diagnostic criteria for polycystic ovary syndrome: towards a rational approach. In: *Polycystic ovary syndrome*, A. Dunaif, J.R. Givens, F.P. Haseltine, & G.R. Merriam, (Eds.), Blackwell, ISBN 0-86542-142-0, Boston, U.S.A. Ch. 32, pp. 377-384

6

Association of Gestational Diabetes Mellitus in Women with Polycystic Ovary Syndrome and Evaluation of Role of Metformin in Reducing the Risk

Fauzia Haq Nawaz and Tahira Naru
Aga Khan University Hospital
Pakistan

1. Introduction

1.1 Objective

To evaluate the prevalence of gestational diabetes mellitus (GDM) in women with polycystic ovary syndrome (PCOS) and to investigate the efficacy of Metformin in reduction of gestational diabetes in women with polycystic ovary syndrome.

1.2 Design

Review of literature on prevalence of gestational diabetes and evaluation of efficacy of Metformin in reducing the prevalence of gestational diabetes in women with polycystic ovary syndrome.

1.3 Setting

Reproductive Endocrinology section of Department of Obstetrics and Gynecology of Aga Khan University Hospital Karachi Pakistan.

1.4 Patient(s)

Women with PCOS and gestational diabetes

1.5 Intervention(s)

Literature search in the electronic databases MEDLINE, study of the references of all relevant trials or reviews, and manual search of the abstracts from the major meetings in the field of human reproduction.

1.6 Main outcome measure

Odds Ratio(OR) for the occurrence of gestational Diabetes.

1.7 Result(s)

Women with PCOS demonstrated a significantly higher risk for the development of GDM as compared with women without PCOS

1.8 Description

The Polycystic Ovarian Syndrome (PCOS) is a common endocrinopathy, affecting approximately 5-10% of women of reproductive age. In its classical form, the syndrome is characterized by oligo- or anovulation, biochemical or clinical hyperandrogenismand polycystic ovarian morphology on ultrasonography. Although much remains unknown regarding the underlying path physiology of PCOS, a form of insulin resistance intrinsic to the syndromeappears to play a central role in its development. Among many women with PCOS, the observed insulin resistance is partially explained by excess adiposity; however, it is increasingly recognized that even lean women with PCOS have increased insulin resistance compared with normal controls. Affected women have an increased risk of glucose intolerance, gestational diabetes mellitus (GDM) and type 2 diabetes. Some, studies suggest the risk of GDM is higher among PCOS versus non-PCOS women, and several studies note an increased prevalence of polycystic ovarian morphology and symptoms in women with prior GDM.

Insulin resistance is defined as the decreased ability of insulin to stimulate glucose disposal into target tissues, or a reduced glucose response to a given amount of insulin. Chronic hyperinsulinemia is a compensatory response to this target tissue resistance. Several mechanisms have been suggested to explain insulin resistance, including peripheral target tissue resistance, decreased hepatic clearance, or increased pancreatic sensitivity. The peripheral insulin resistance in PCOS is uniquely due to a defect beyond the activation of the receptor kinase, namely, reduced tyrosine autophosphorylation of the insulin receptor and enhances the expression of hyperandrogenism by its inhibitory effect on hepatic sex hormone binding globulin (SHBG) production thereby increasing the bioavailability of androgens which leads to metabolic and obstetrical complications. Significant metabolic burden of insulin resistance is seen in women with PCOS, affected women may have an increased risk of impaired glucose tolerance (IGT), GDM and type 2 diabetes mellitus (DM).

In pregnant women with PCOS, the increasing tissue resistance to insulin, mainly caused by placental hormones, adds on the preexisting state of insulin resistance, which may accompany the syndrome. This pathogenic mechanism could lead to hyperglycemia, reflected in a higher incidence of GDM. However, studies on GDM prevalence in women with PCOS gave conflicting results; considering the heterogeneity of PCOS and the diversity in methodology of screening and diagnosing GDM, these results should have been expected.

A method of combining the results of the studies addressing the risk of Incidence of GDM in women with PCOS was one of the endpoints in addressing pregnancy complications in women with PCOS. Women with PCOS demonstrated a significantly higher chance of the development of GDM, though with significant statistical heterogeneity among the studies. This heterogeneity was not further analyzed or accounted for. To examine whether women with PCOS have a greater risk for the development of GDM than women without PCOS, we performed a review of literature and analysis of available trial

2. PCOS, Gestational Diabetes Mellitus (GDM) and diabetes

It has been recognized that women with PCOS have a higher risk for developing type 2 diabetes mellitus and gestational diabetes .In a retrospective cohort follow-up of patients with PCOS, the prevalence of diabetes mellitus was 7-fold higher than in controls.

Gestational diabetes is defined as impaired glucose tolerance diagnosed for the first time during pregnancy, occurs in 2-5% of pregnancies and usually resolves at the end of gestation. However, between one half and one third of women with gestational diabetes may develop diabetes 2-11 years post-partum. Different studies have shown that women with PCOS have a higher risk for the development of gestational diabetes in relation to insulin resistance . Moreover, other authors have demonstrated a high incidence of polycystic ovaries in women with history of gestational diabetes Gestational diabetes is associated with a high neonatal morbidity and given that patients with PCOS have a high prevalence of gestational diabetes, these women should be considered to be at risk. Therefore, preventive measures before pregnancy to minimize neonatal morbidity should be recommended, including dietary advice and physical exercise as well as to indicate insulin-sensitizing treatments before; and during pregnancy.

In reproductive age, the prevalence of type 2 diabetes mellitus is estimated between 1.7 and 6.1%. This prevalence would be expected to be from 5-10-fold higher in women with PCOS. On the other hand, PCOS may be considered a pre-diabetic state with a prevalence of impaired glucose tolerance of 31-35% and a prevalence of type 2 diabetes of 7.5-10%. Impaired glucose tolerance is characterized by moderate increases of fasting glucose levels that may precede diabetes. Women with impaired glucose tolerance are asymptomatic; therefore, an oral glucose tolerance test is required for diagnosis. Conversion of impaired glucose tolerance to frank diabetes in women with PCOS is 5-10 times more frequent compared with normal women The mean age at diagnosis of type 2 diabetes mellitus in patients with PCOS (30-40 years of age) is lower than in normal women (60-70 years of age) Additionally, a family history of diabetes and the presence of obesity are important predictors for the development of type 2 diabetes mellitus.

The diagnostic criteria of diabetes based on the 1999 World Health Organization definition and the 1997 recommendations of the Expert Committee of the ADA is a fasting glucose level ≥126mg/dl (7mmol/l) or oral glucose tolerance test (2h plasma glucose after 75g oral glucose challenge) ≥200mg/dl (11.1mmol/l). Diagnostic criteria of impaired glucose tolerance include normal fasting glucose levels (<126mg/dl) in association with oral glucose tolerance test ≥140 and <200mg/dl (7.8-11.1mmol/l). Normal baseline plasma glucose levels are 110mg/dl (6.1mmol/l). The principal difference between the 1997 ADA criteria and the 1999 WHO criteria is that the ADA criteria discourage the use of the oral glucose tolerance test as a routine diagnostic tool whereas the WHO criteria do not. However, it seems that the WHO criteria are more adequate for the diagnosis of diabetes in women with PCOS tolerance test .

These data indicate that women with PCOS are at high risk for long-term development of type 2 diabetes mellitus, and support the importance of an early diagnosis and treatment of insulin resistance to help reduce the incidence and severity of diabetes, dyslipidemia, hypertension and cardiovascular disease

3. Review of role of insulin sensitizing agents (metformin) in prevention of gestational diabetes in women with pcos

A major change in the treatment of PCOS was initiated by the understanding that many women with this disorder compensate insulin resistance with a period of hyper secretion of insulin by the pancreatic beta cell. This understanding has been incorporated into the framework of PCOS treatments through the beneficial effects of insulin-sensitizing treatments on the PCOS phenotype Agents that improve insulin sensitivity (and lower circulating insulin levels) include metformin as well as thiazolidinediones, pioglitazone and rosiglitazone as alternative pharmacotherapies for those who cannot tolerate metformin as a result of gastrointestinal side effects .These treatments have resulted in beneficial changes in PCOS phenotype with increased menstrual and ovulatory frequency, pregnancy and decreased hirsutism. On the other hand, an increase in obstetrical pathology in women with PCOS has been documented, including increased rates of miscarriage, gestational diabetes, macrosomia, caesarean deliveries and pre-eclampsia. Given that hyperinsulinaemia may play a role in the pathophysiology of these conditions, maintenance of oral antidiabetic agents during pregnancy may decrease the incidence of these complications. Metformin, with a high safety profile for use during pregnancy, has been given to pregnant women with PCOS resulting in a reduction of the aforementioned conditions in these patients.

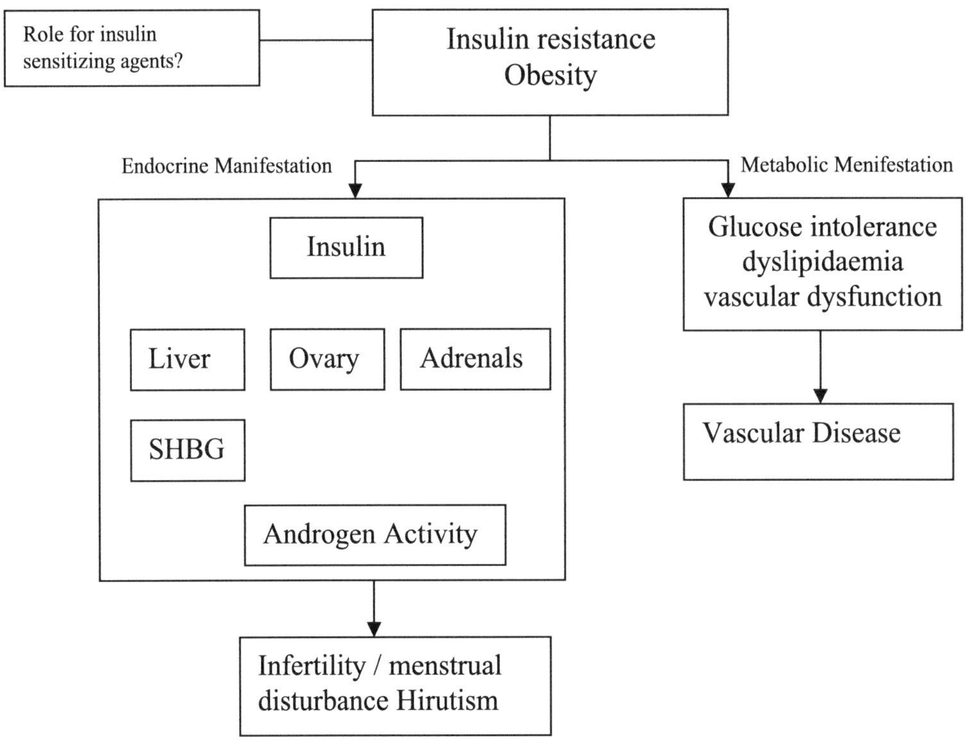

Fig. 1. Postulated role for insulin sensitizing agents on target tissues affected in woman with PCOS Harborne L etal

These concepts have quickly become the cornerstone of diagnosis and treatment of PCOS and other diseases also associated with insulin resistance. Type 2 diabetes mellitus and gestational diabetes. Recent observations regarding the effect of insulin-sensitizing drugs on ovarian stimulation in patients with PCOS undergoing IVF are also discussed, as well as the current status of the use of insulin-sensitizing drugs during pregnancy. Finally, substantial progress has been made to elucidate the cellular and molecular mechanisms of insulin resistance in PCOS. The insulin receptor and genetics of PCOS are complex areas that are extensively being investigated.

These agents increase the tissue sensitivity to insulin action in vivo .The agent commonly used in clinical practice is metformin, an oral hypoglycemic biguanide. Newer agents include the thiazolidinediones group of drugs like troglitazone. Hepatotoxocity of this drug has lead to its withdrawal, but pioglitazone and D-chiroinositol has been used with some success in an insulin sensitization in women with PCOS

3.1 Metformin

It acts primarily by increasing peripheral glucose uptake in response to insulin at post receptor level, with some basal reduction in gluconeogenesis. It improves the insulin sensitivity in adipose tissues and skeletal muscles. All of the action are mediated by CAMP activated by protein kinase .It has been suggested that various insulin sensitizing drugs specifically inhibits the 17 , 20 lyase activity of P450c 17 . While it true that these drugs lower the C19 steroids but still the exact mechanism of action of metformin is not clear.

Until now the use of insulin sensitizing agents are targeted toward symptoms and signs of PCOS, like in ovulation induction, as an anti androgen therapy and for hirsutism. In this chapter we will be discussing the role of insulin sensitizers particularly metformin in prevention of Gestational diabetes associated with PCOS in light of recent evidence support.

3.2 Use of metformin and prevention and treatment of gestational diabetes mellitus

Metformin has been used to treat diabetes in second and third trimesters of pregnancy after the main teratogenic period, no significant perinatal morbidity and mortality was noticed except relatively high frequency of neonatal jaundice. Coetzee *et al.*14, has published the experience of 118 pregnant women with PCOS, who received an oral hypoglycemic medication and found the higher frequency of preeclampsia and perinatal mortality. However when these study results were critically analyzed it was found these women were older, more obese than their reference group which accounted for the baseline characteristics rather than Metformin alone.

The incidence of gestational diabetes in women with PCOS appears to be increased but data are not consistent .Insulin resistance in PCOS and the inability of pancreatic beta cells to compensate for increased needs of insulin during pregnancy are risk factors for gestational diabetes.

Different studies have documented a decrease in the incidence of gestational diabetes in PCOS women treated with metformin during pregnancy. Although in most of them retrospective controls were used. Prospective randomized studies with a sufficient number of patients are necessary in order to provide good evidence to recommend the use of metformin during pregnancy.

4. Conclusion

PCOS is one of the most common hormonal disorder affecting women and has reproductive, metabolic, cardiovascular health implications across the life span. Insulin resistance in PCOS has been considered as main etiological factor for major health related consequences. Significant heterogeneity among studies and dependence of the outcome on study type make the higher risk of GDM in women with PCOS a questionable finding. The conduction of properly designed studies should precede any recommendation to pregnant women with PCOS in regard to the risk of GDM.

5. Refrences

[1] 1997 Report of the Expert Committee on the Diagnosis and Classification of Diabetes Mellitus. Diabetes Care 20:1183-1197

[2] 1998 Will new diagnostic criteria for diabetes mellitus change phenotype of patients with diabetes? Reanalysis of European epidemiological data. DECODE Study Group on behalf of the European Diabetes Epidemiology Study Group. BMJ 317:371-375

[3] American Association of Clinical Endocrinologists Polycystic Ovary Syndrome Writing Committee 2005 American Association of Clinical Endocrinologists Position Statement on Metabolic and Cardiovascular Consequences of Polycystic Ovary Syndrome. Endocr Pract 11:126-134

[4] American Diabetes Association 2007 Standards of medical care in diabetes-2007. Diabetes Care 30(Suppl 1):S4-S41

[5] American Diabetes Association 2007 Standards of medical care in diabetes-2007. Diabetes Care 30(Suppl 1):S4-S41

[6] Arslanian SA, Lewy V, Danadian K, Saad R 2002 Metformin therapy in obese adolescents with polycystic ovary syndrome and impaired glucose tolerance: amelioration of exaggerated adrenal response to adrenocorticotropin with reduction of insulinemia/insulin resistance. J Clin Endocrinol Metab 87:1555-1559

[7] Arslanian SA, Lewy VD, Danadian K 2001 Glucose intolerance in obese adolescents with polycystic ovary syndrome: roles of insulin resistance and β-cell dysfunction and risk of cardiovascular disease. J Clin Endocrinol Metab 86:66-71

[8] Asuncion M, Calvo RM, San Millan JL, Sancho J, Avila S, Escobar-Morreale HF 2000 A prospective study of the prevalence of the polycystic ovary syndrome in unselected Caucasian women from Spain. J Clin Endocrinol Metab 85:2434-2438

[9] Azziz R, Carmina E, Dewailly D, Diamanti-Kandarakis E, Escobar-Morreale HF, Futterweit W, Janssen OE, Legro RS, Norman RJ, Taylor AE, Witchel SF, Androgen Excess Society 2006 Positions statement: criteria for defining polycystic ovary syndrome as a predominantly hyperandrogenic syndrome: an Androgen Excess Society guideline. J Clin Endocrinol Metab 91:4237-4245

[10] Azziz R, Woods KS, Reyna R, Key TJ, Knochenhauer ES, Yildiz BO 2004 The prevalence and features of the polycystic ovary syndrome in an unselected population. J Clin Endocrinol Metab 89:2745-2749

[11] Baillargeon JP, Diamanti-Kandarakis E, Ostlund Jr RE, Apridonidze T, Iuorno MJ, Nestler JE 2006 Altered D-chiro-inositol urinary clearance in women with polycystic ovary syndrome. Diabetes Care 29:300-305

[12] Baillargeon JP, Iuorno MJ, Jakubowicz DJ, Apridonidze T, He N, Nestler JE 2004 Metformin therapy increases insulin-stimulated release of D-chiro-inositol-containing inositolphosphoglycan mediator in women with polycystic ovary syndrome. J Clin Endocrinol Metab 89:242-249

[13] Barrett-Connor E, Ferrara A 1998 Isolated postchallenge hyperglycemia and the risk of fatal cardiovascular disease in older women and men. The Rancho Bernardo Study. Diabetes Care 21:1236-1239

[14] Boomsma CM, Eijkemans MJ, Hughes EG, Visser GH, Fauser BC, Macklon NS 2006 A meta-analysis of pregnancy outcomes in women with polycystic ovary syndrome. Hum Reprod Update 12:673-683

[15] Bridger T, MacDonald S, Baltzer F, Rodd C 2006 Randomized placebo-controlled trial of metformin for adolescents with polycystic ovary syndrome. Arch Pediatr Adolesc Med 160:241-246

[16] Centers for Disease Control and Prevention (CDC) 2003 Prevalence of diabetes and impaired fasting glucose in adults-United States, 1999-2000. MMWR Morb Mortal Wkly Rep 52:833-837

[17] Chen X, Yang D, Li L, Feng S, Wang L 2006 Abnormal glucose tolerance in Chinese women with polycystic ovary syndrome. Hum Reprod 21:2027-2032

[18] Chiasson JL, Josse RG, Gomis R, Hanefeld M, Karasik A, Laakso M 2002 Acarbose for prevention of type 2 diabetes mellitus: the STOP-NIDDM randomised trial. Lancet 359:2072-2077

[19] Coetzee EJ and Jackson WP .Oral hypoglycemic in the first trimester and fetal out come .S Afr Med J 1984; 65: 635-637

[20] Denburg MR, Manibo AM, Lobo RA, Jaffe R, Ferin M, Levine LS, Oberfield SE 2003 Early endocrine, metabolic, and sonographic characteristics of polycystic ovary syndrome (PCOS): comparison between nonobese and obese adolescents. J Clin Endocrinol Metab 88:4682-4688

[21] Dereli D, Dereli T, Bayraktar F, Ozgen AG, Yilmaz C 2005 Endocrine and metabolic effects of rosiglitazone in non-obese women with polycystic ovary disease. Endocr J 52:299-308

[22] Diabetes Prevention Program Research Group 2003 Effects of withdrawal from metformin on the development of diabetes in the diabetes prevention program. Diabetes Care 26:977-980

[23] Diamanti-Kandarakis E, Kouli CR, Bergiele AT, Filandra FA, Tsianateli TC, Spina GG, Zapanti ED, Bartzis MI 1999 A survey of the polycystic ovary syndrome in the Greek island of Lesbos: hormonal and metabolic profile. J Clin Endocrinol Metab 84:4006-4011

[24] Dunaif A, Finegood DT 1996 β-Cell dysfunction independent of obesity and glucose intolerance in the polycystic ovary syndrome. J Clin Endocrinol Metab 81:942-947

[25] Dunaif A, Segal KR, Futterweit W, Dobrjansky A 1989 Profound peripheral insulin resistance, independent of obesity, in polycystic ovary syndrome. Diabetes 38:1165–1174
[26] Dunaif A, Segal KR, Shelley DR, Green G, Dobrjansky A, Licholai T 1992 Evidence for distinctive and intrinsic defects in insulin action in polycystic ovary syndrome. Diabetes 41:1257–1266
[27] Durbin RJ 2004 Thiazolidinedione therapy in the prevention/delay of type 2 diabetes in patients with impaired glucose tolerance and insulin resistance. Diabetes Obes Metab 6:280–285
[28] Ehrmann DA 2000 Glucose intolerance in the polycystic ovary syndrome: role of the pancreatic β-cell. J Pediatr Endocrinol Metab 13(Suppl 5):1299–1301
[29] Ehrmann DA, Barnes RB, Rosenfield RL, Cavaghan MK, Imperial J 1999 Prevalence of impaired glucose tolerance and diabetes in women with polycystic ovary syndrome. Diabetes Care 22:141–146
[30] Ehrmann DA, Kasza K, Azziz R, Legro RS, Ghazzi MN 2005 Effects of race and family history of type 2 diabetes on metabolic status of women with polycystic ovary syndrome. J Clin Endocrinol Metab 90:66–71
[31] Ek I, Arner P, Bergqvist A, Carlstrom K, Wahrenberg H 1997 Impaired adipocyte lipolysis in nonobese women with the polycystic ovary syndrome: a possible link to insulin resistance? J Clin Endocrinol Metab 82:1147–1153
[32] Ek I, Arner P, Ryden M, Holm C, Thörne A, Hoffstedt J, Wahrenberg H 2002 A unique defect in the regulation of visceral fat cell lipolysis in the polycystic ovary syndrome as an early link to insulin resistance. Diabetes 51:484–492
[33] Expert Panel on Detection, Evaluation, and Treatment of High Blood Cholesterol in Adults 2001 Executive Summary of The Third Report of The National Cholesterol Education Program (NCEP) Expert Panel on Detection, Evaluation, And Treatment of High Blood Cholesterol In Adults (Adult Treatment Panel III). JAMA 285:2486–2497
[34] Gabir MM, Hanson RL, Dabelea D, Imperatore G, Roumain J, Bennett PH, Knowler WC 2000 The 1997 American Diabetes Association and 1999 World Health Organization criteria for hyperglycemia in the diagnosis and prediction of diabetes. Diabetes Care 23:1108–1112
[35] Gerstein HC, Yusuf S, Bosch J, Pogue J, Sheridan P, Dinccag N, Hanefeld M, Hoogwerf B, Laakso M, Mohan V, Shaw J, Zinman B, Holman RR 2006 Effect of rosiglitazone on the frequency of diabetes in patients with impaired glucose tolerance or impaired fasting glucose: a randomised controlled trial. Lancet 368:1096–1105
[36] Goodarzi MO, Erickson S, Port SC, Jennrich RI, Korenman SG 2005 β-Cell function: a key pathological determinant in polycystic ovary syndrome. J Clin Endocrinol Metab 90:310–315
[37] Heymsfield SB, Segal KR, Hauptman J, Lucas CP, Boldrin MN, Rissanen A, Wilding JP, Sjöström L 2000 Effects of weight loss with orlistat on glucose tolerance and progression to type 2 diabetes in obese adults. Arch Intern Med 160:1321–1326

[38] Holte J, Gennarelli G, Wide L, Lithell H, Berne C 1998 High prevalence of polycystic ovaries and associated clinical, endocrine, and metabolic features in women with previous gestational diabetes mellitus. J Clin Endocrinol Metab 83:1143–1150

[39] Ibanez L, Potau N, Marcos MV, de Zegher F 2000 Treatment of hirsutism, hyperandrogenism, oligomenorrhea, dyslipidemia, and hyperinsulinism in nonobese, adolescent girls: effect of flutamide. J Clin Endocrinol Metab 85:3251–3255Silfen ME,

[40] Kaneko T, Wang PY, Tawata M, Sato 1998 A low carbohydrate intake before oral glucose-tolerance tests. Lancet 352:289

[41] Kinoshita T, Kato J 1990 Impaired glucose tolerance in patients with polycystic ovary syndrome (PCOS). Horm Res 33(Suppl 2):18–20

[42] Knochenhauer ES, Key TJ, Kahsar-Miller M, Waggoner W, Boots LR, Azziz R 1998 Prevalence of the polycystic ovary syndrome in unselected black and white women of the southeastern United States: a prospective study. J Clin Endocrinol Metab 83:3078–3082

[43] Knowler WC, Barrett-Connor E, Fowler SE, Hamman RF, Lachin JM, Walker EA, Nathan DM, Diabetes Prevention Program Research Group 2002 Reduction in the incidence of type 2 diabetes with lifestyle intervention or metformin. N Engl J Med 346:393–403

[44] Knowler WC, Hamman RF, Edelstein SL, Barrett-Connor E, Ehrmann DA, Walker EA, Fowler SE, Nathan DM, Kahn SE, Diabetes Prevention Program Research Group 2005 Prevention of type 2 diabetes with troglitazone in the Diabetes Prevention Program. Diabetes 54:1150–1156

[45] Koivunen RM, Juutinen J, Vauhkonen I, Morin-Papunen LC, Roukonen A, Tapanainen JS 2001 Metabolic and steroidogenic alterations related to increased frequency of polycystic ovaries in women with a history of gestational diabetes. J Clin Endocrinol Metab 86:2591–2599

[46] Kurioka H, Takahashi K, Miyazaki K 2007 Glucose intolerance in Japanese patients with polycystic ovary syndrome. Arch Gynecol Obstet 275:169–173

[47] Legro RS, Castracane VD, Kauffman RP 2004 Detecting insulin resistance in polycystic ovary syndrome: purposes and pitfalls. Obstet Gynecol Surv 59:141–154

[48] Legro RS, Gnatuk CL, Kunselman AR, Dunaif A 2005 Changes in glucose tolerance over time in women with polycystic ovary syndrome: a controlled study. J Clin Endocrinol Metab 90:3236–3242Anttila L, Karjala K, Penttila RA, Ruutiainen K, Ekblad U 1998 Polycystic ovaries in women with gestational diabetes. Obstet Gynecol 92:13–16

[49] Legro RS, Kunselman AR, Dodson WC, Dunaif A 1999 Prevalence and predictors of risk for type 2 diabetes mellitus and impaired glucose tolerance in polycystic ovary syndrome: a prospective, controlled study in 254 affected women. J Clin Endocrinol Metab 84:165–169

[50] Lo JC, Feigenbaum SL, Escobar GJ, Yang J, Crites YM, Ferrara A 2006 Increased prevalence of gestational diabetes mellitus among women with diagnosed

polycystic ovary syndrome: a population-based study. Diabetes Care 29:1915-1917

[51] Moghetti P, Castello R, Negri C, Tosi F, Perrone F, Caputo M, Zanolin E, Muggeo M 2000 Metformin effects on clinical features, endocrine and metabolic profiles, and insulin sensitivity in polycystic ovary syndrome: a randomized, double-blind, placebo-controlled 6-month trial, followed by open, long-term clinical evaluation. J Clin Endocrinol Metab 85:139-146

[52] Mohlig M, Floter A, Spranger J, Weickert MO, Schill T, Schlösser HW, Brabant G, Pfeiffer AF, Selbig J, Schöfl C 2006 Predicting impaired glucose metabolism in women with polycystic ovary syndrome by decision tree modelling. Diabetologia 49:2572-2579

[53] Nestler JE, Jakubowicz DJ, Reamer P, Gunn RD, Allan G 1999 Ovulatory and metabolic effects of D-chiro-inositol in the polycystic ovary syndrome. N Engl J Med 340:1314-1320

[54] Nestler JE, Sharma ST, Misleading effects of a low-carbohydrate diet on glucose intolerance testing in women with PCOS: a case report. Program of the 88th Annual Meeting of The Endocrine Society, Boston, MA, 2006, p 857 (Abstract P3-844)

[55] Norman RJ, Mahabeer S, Masters S 1995 Ethnic differences in insulin and glucose response to glucose between white and Indian women with polycystic ovary syndrome. Fertil Steril 63:58-62

[56] Norman RJ, Masters L, Milner CR, Wang JX, Davies MJ 2001 Relative risk of conversion from normoglycaemia to impaired glucose tolerance or non-insulin dependent diabetes mellitus in polycystic ovarian syndrome. Hum Reprod 16:1995-1998

[57] Palmert MR, Gordon CM, Kartashov AI, Legro RS, Emans SJ, Dunaif A 2002 Screening for abnormal glucose tolerance in adolescents with polycystic ovary syndrome. J Clin Endocrinol Metab 87:1017-1023

[58] Pan XR, Li GW, Hu YH, Wang JX, Yang WY, An ZX, Hu ZX, Lin J, Xiao JZ, Cao HB, Liu PA, Jiang XG, Jiang YY, Wang JP, Zheng H, Zhang H, Bennett PH, Howard BV 1997 Effects of diet and exercise in preventing NIDDM in people with impaired glucose tolerance. The Da Qing IGT and Diabetes Study. Diabetes Care 20:537-544

[59] Ramachandran A, Snehalatha C, Mary S, Mukesh B, Bhaskar AD, Vijay V 2006 The Indian Diabetes Prevention Programme shows that lifestyle modification and metformin prevent type 2 diabetes in Asian Indian subjects with impaired glucose tolerance (IDPP-1). Diabetologia 49:289-297

[60] Rosenbaum D, Haber RS, Dunaif A 1993 Insulin resistance in polycystic ovary syndrome: decreased expression of GLUT-4 glucose transporters in adipocytes. Am J Physiol 264(2 Pt 1):E197-E202

[61] Rotterdam ESHRE/ASRM-Sponsored PCOS Consensus Workshop Group 2004 Revised 2003 consensus on diagnostic criteria and long-term health risks related to polycystic ovary syndrome. Fertil Steril 81:19-25

[62] Saad R, Gungor N, Arslanian S 2005 Progression from normal glucose tolerance to type 2 diabetes in a young girl: longitudinal changes in insulin sensitivity and secretion assessed by the clamp technique and surrogate estimates. Pediatr Diabetes 6:95–99

[63] Sharma ST, Nestler JE 2006 Prevention of diabetes and cardiovascular disease in women with PCOS: treatment with insulin sensitizers. Best Pract Res Clin Endocrinol Metab 20:245–260

[64] Soderberg S, Zimmet P, Tuomilehto J, de Courten M, Dowse GK, Chitson P, Stenlund H, Gareeboo H, Alberti KG, Shaw J 2004 High incidence of type 2 diabetes and increasing conversion rates from impaired fasting glucose and impaired glucose tolerance to diabetes in Mauritius. J Intern Med 256:37–47

[65] The DREAM Trial Investigators 2006 Effect of ramipril on the incidence of diabetes. N Engl J Med 355:1551–1562

[66] The Rotterdam ESHRE/ASRM-Sponsored PCOS Consensus Workshop Group 2004 Revised 2003 consensus on diagnostic criteria and long-term health risks related to polycystic ovary syndrome (PCOS). Hum Reprod 19:41–47

[67] Tominaga M, Eguchi H, Manaka H, Igarashi K, Kato T, Sekikawa A 1999 Impaired glucose tolerance is a risk factor for cardiovascular disease, but not impaired fasting glucose. The Funagata Diabetes Study. Diabetes Care 22:920–924

[68] Torgerson JS, Hauptman J, Boldrin MN, Sjostrom L 2004 XENical in the prevention of diabetes in obese subjects (XENDOS) study: a randomized study of orlistat as an adjunct to lifestyle changes for the prevention of type 2 diabetes in obese patients. Diabetes Care 27:155–161

[69] Trolle B, Lauszus FF 2005 Risk factors for glucose intolerance in Danish women with polycystic ovary syndrome. Acta Obstet Gynecol Scand 84:1192–1196

[70] Tuomilehto J, Lindstrom J, Eriksson JG, Valle TT, Hämäläinen H, Ilanne-Parikka P, Keinänen-Kiukaanniemi S, Laakso M, Louheranta A, Rastas M, Salminen V, Uusitupa M, Finnish Diabetes Prevention Study Group 2001 Prevention of type 2 diabetes mellitus by changes in lifestyle among subjects with impaired glucose tolerance. N Engl J Med 344:1343–1350

[71] Unluhizarci K, Kelestimur F, Bayram F, Sahin Y, Tutus A 1999 The effects of metformin on insulin resistance and ovarian steroidogenesis in women with polycystic ovary syndrome. Clin Endocrinol (Oxf) 51:231–236

[72] Vrbikova J, Dvorakova K, Grimmichova T, Hill M, Stanicka S, Cibula D, Bendlova B, Starka L, Vondra K 2007 Prevalence of insulin resistance and prediction of glucose intolerance and type 2 diabetes mellitus in women with polycystic ovary syndrome. Clin Chem Lab Med 45:639–644

[73] Weerakiet S, Srisombut C, Bunnag P, Sangtong S, Chuangsoongnoen N, Rojanasakul A 2001 Prevalence of type 2 diabetes mellitus and impaired glucose tolerance in Asian women with polycystic ovary syndrome. Int J Gynaecol Obstet 75:177–184

[74] Wein P, Beischer N, Harris C, Permezel M 1999 A trial of simple versus intensified dietary modification for prevention of progression to diabetes mellitus in women with impaired glucose tolerance. Aust N Z J Obstet Gynaecol 39:162–166

[75] WHO Study Group on Diabetes Mellitus 1985 Diabetes mellitus: report of a WHO study group. Geneva: World Health Organization
[76] Wing RR, Venditti E, Jakicic JM, Polley BA, Lang W 1998 Lifestyle intervention in overweight individuals with a family history of diabetes. Diabetes Care 21:350-359
[77] World Health Organization 2006 Definition and diagnosis of diabetes mellitus and intermediate hyperglycemia: report of a WHO/IDF consultation. Geneva: World Health Organization

7

Polycystic Ovary Syndrome and Cardiovascular Disease

Barış Önder Pamuk[1], Derun Taner Ertugrul[2], Hamiyet Yılmaz[3] and M. Muzaffer İlhan[4]
[1]*İzmir Bozyaka Research and Training Hospital, Department of Internal Medicine*
[2]*Kecioren Research and Training Hospital, Department of Internal Medicine*
[3]*Aydin State Hospital, Department of Internal Medicine*
[4]*Ege University Medical School, Department of Internal Medicine*
Turkey

1. Introduction

Young women have an inferior risk of cardiac events, but this benefit fades after menopause, leaving them at risk to develop a cardiovascular disease (CVD) (Stramba-Badiale, Fox et al. 2006). Endocrine and gynecologic diseases may have impact on this pattern. Ever since the classical notice of Stein and Leventhal in 1935 (Stein and Leventhal. 1935), interest in polycystic ovaries (PCO) and its accompanying syndrome (PCOS) has grown from a ''gynecological curiosity to a multisystem endocrinopathy'' (Homburg 1996). Actually, polycystic ovary syndrome (PCOS), is the most common female endocrinopathy in up to 10% in reproductive age and appears to be related with an increased cardiovascular risk (Talbott, Guzick et al. 1995; Cibula, Cifkova et al. 2000). The syndrome is characterized by chronic anovulation and hyperandrogenism (Franks 1995; Scarpitta and Sinagra 2000). Cardiovascular disease and type 2 diabetes are two potential major long-term sequelae of this condition that is worth of examination.

Even though the first description occurred almost 70 years ago, there has not been agreement about its definition. At a recent collective European Society of Human Reproduction and Embryology/American Society for Reproductive Medicine (ESHRE/ASRM) consensus meeting, a refined definition of PCOS was agreed: particularly, the presence of two out of the following three criteria:

i. oligo- and/or anovulation
ii. hyperandrogenism (clinical and/or biochemical)
iii. polycystic ovaries, with the exclusion of other etiologies (2004).

It is widely accepted that polycystic ovary syndrome (PCOS) is correlated with an increased risk of cardiovascular disease. Dyslipidaemia (Legro, Kunselman et al. 2001; Pirwany, Fleming et al. 2001), hypertension (Dahlgren, Janson et al. 1992; Luque-Ramirez, Alvarez-Blasco et al. 2007) and diabetes (Ehrmann, Barnes et al. 1999; Legro, Kunselman et al. 1999) are appeared to be more common in women with PCOS. Obesity, especially central obesity, is a pivotal factor for predicting the long-term risk of cardiovascular disease (Franks, Kiddy et al. 1991; Luque-Ramirez, Alvarez-Blasco et al. 2007). There is substantial convergence among these features found in PCOS and the metabolic syndrome, and it is potential that these are interrelated conditions. Alterations in clotting (Manneras-Holm, Baghaei et al. 2011) and blood vessel function (Paradisi, Steinberg et al. 2001) might describe why cardiovascular disease is a long-term risk in women with PCOS.

However metabolic abnormalities aforementioned and obesity were not recognized until reduced sensitivity to insulin and compensatory hyperinsulinemia were demonstrated in PCOS patients. The metabolic profile well known in women with PCOS, is equivalent to the insulin resistance syndrome, a clustering within an individual with hyperinsulinemia, mild glucose intolerance, dyslipidemia, and hypertension. The insulin resistance syndrome (or syndrome X) has been recognized as a risk factor for developing type 2 diabetes and CVD (Legro, Kunselman et al. 1999; Korhonen, Hippelainen et al. 2001).

There is also a strong association between hyperandrogenemia and insulin resistance in PCOS (Bremer and Miller 2008). This may mainly consider the stimulatory effect of hyperinsulinemia on ovarian androgen production, although hyperandrogenemia may finally contribute to insulin resistance (Baptiste, Battista et al. 2010). This may also underlie the association between hyperandrogenemia and impaired vascular function and reported in some studies involving PCOS subjects (Wu and von Eckardstein 2003). Nevertheless, even though insulin resistance per se has been associated with endothelial dysfunction and increased cardiovascular risk, there is no stable proof that hyperandrogenemia is a risk factor for cardiovascular disease in women (Gorgels, v d Graaf et al. 1997).

Notwithstanding the fact that PCOS is increasingly recognized as being associated with a cluster of cardiovascular risk factors, there is no final evidence for increased cardiovascular events in PCOS. Nor is there, evidently, data show that PCOS alone imparts increased risk independent of associated risk factors. This article intends to review the spectrum of cardiovascular risk factors, the cardiovascular epidemiology and especially the most recent studies of subclinical cardiovascular disease in PCOS, investigating cardiovascular structure and function. Although, these latter sets of studies have, in particular, further elucidated the causal links between PCOS and cardiovascular disease.

2. Cardiovascular risk factors in PCOS

2.1 Biochemical

2.1.1 Hyperinsulinemia and insulin resistance

Insulin resistance, described as a reduced glucose response to a given amount of insulin, is a typical metabolic disturbance related with PCOS. Resistance to the activity of insulin in target tissues is a main pathogenic factor in metabolic syndrome and type 2 diabetes. Association of PCOS with insulin resistance was known nearly three decades ago (Burghen, Givens et al. 1980). Hyperinsulinemic euglycemic clamp measurements have shown that insulin-mediated glucose uptake have decreased by 35-40% in both lean and obese women with PCOS, similar to the degree of insulin resistance seen in patients with type 2 diabetes (Dunaif, Segal et al. 1989). Insulin resistance causes compensatory hyperinsulinemia, which is related to many of the phenotypic features of PCOS (menstrual disturbances, evolvement of ovarian cysts, hirsutism and other associated disorders) through multiple mechanisms, involving ovarian steroidogenesis, gonadotrophin secretion, and sex hormone binding globulin production (Ehrmann 2005). Insulin can enhance ovarian steroidogenesis and enhance directly, independently and/or augment LH-mediated androgen production (Barbieri, Makris et al. 1984; Poretsky, Cataldo et al. 1999; Bremer and Miller 2008). Hence, hyperinsulinemia and hyperandrogenemia are two essential characteristics of PCOS. Their cause and effect relationship is still debated (Dunaif 1997; Poretsky, Cataldo et al. 1999; Legro, Gnatuk et al. 2005; Bremer and Miller 2008). However, several evidences suggest that hyperinsulinemia may be the principal cause leading to the ovarian hyperandrogenemia. Insulin level reduction pharmacologically, has been ameliorating hyperinsulinemia as well as hyperandrogenemia and restore ovulation in the women with PCOS. Even though, a decrease in androgen levels by bilateral oophorectomy, administration of GnRH agonist (Bremer and Miller 2008), or antiandrogenic combinations (Dunaif 1997) had no impact on IR or hyperinsulinemia in the PCOS women, which would have been expected if hyperandrogenemia was the factor of hyperinsulinemia. Besides, the peripheral insulin resistance in PCOS was related to defective pancreatic ß-cell function (Ehrmann, Sturis et al. 1995). Additionally, insulin resistance increases the risk for evolvement of glucose intolerance, type 2 diabetes mellitus (T2DM), hypertension, dyslipidemia and cardiovascular abnormalities in these patients (Maitra, Pingle et al. 2001; Legro, Gnatuk et al. 2005).

PCOS patients have a higher incidence of insulin resistance and hyperinsulinemia than age-matched controls in both obese and nonobese patients. Nonetheless, obese women with PCOS have significantly decreased insulin sensitivity compared with nonobese women who have PCOS. Insulin resistance has been known to lead to the progression of type 2 diabetes mellitus. PCOS patients have progress to impaired glucose tolerance in 30% to 40% of the cases, and as many as 10% of them develop type 2 diabetes mellitus by the age of 40 (Clayton, Ogden et al. 1992; Guzick 2004; Tsilchorozidou, Overton et al. 2004). Strong association between insulin resistance and hyperandrogemia has been shown by several studies. This association was first reported by Achard and Thiers in 1921 in a bearded woman who was also a diabetic (Guzick 2004). Androgen production is magnified synergistically with LH and insulin action in the ovarian theca cells. In addition insulin decreases hepatic synthesis and release of sex hormone-binding globulin, the hormone that binds testosterone in the blood flow, hence increasing the amount of free testosterone that is biologically attainable (Tsilchorozidou, Overton et al. 2004). Free testosterone levels typically have been increased in hyperinsulinemic PCOS patients. Although the total testosterone concentration may be at the upper range of normal or only moderately elevated (Tsilchorozidou, Overton et al. 2004).The exact cellular and molecular mechanisms of insulin resistance in PCOS remain elusive in spite of the crucial role of insulin resistance in the pathogenesis of this syndrome. Together intrinsic and acquired defects in insulin signaling, have been known as mediators of insulin resistance in women with PCOS.

In PCOS the "central paradox" is characterized by responsive ovaries to insulin effect to produce androgens in spite of systemic insulin resistant state; nonetheless, classical target organs of insulin as well as ovary remains resistant to its metabolic activity. Distinct insulin target tissues and ovary have comprised optimal number and affinity of insulin receptors, and as well as no structural and mutational abnormalities could be detected in the PCOS women (Dunaif 1997; Ciaraldi, Morales et al. 1998; Book and Dunaif 1999; Poretsky, Cataldo et al. 1999). Therefore, a post-receptor binding defect in the insulin signaling pathway appears to play a consequential function in the etiology of selective IR. Notwithstanding the fact that several in vitro and in vivo researches have been carried out in various tissues to illuminate the possible mechanism of IR and hyperandrogenemia (ovarian cells) (Ovarian cells, adipocytes, fibroblasts, myocytes) (Dunaif 1997; Poretsky, Cataldo et al. 1999; Pessin and Saltiel 2000; Nelson-Degrave, Wickenheisser et al. 2005; Diamanti-Kandarakis and Papavassiliou 2006) in PCOS patients, however the data has not been yet conclusive.

Pancreatic β-cell dysfunction has been described in women with PCOS, whereby there is augmented basal secretion of insulin in spite of an insufficient postprandial response (Ehrmann, Sturis et al. 1995). This imperfection remains even after weight loss, despite an amelioration in glucose tolerance (Holte, Bergh et al. 1995). Insulin performs its effects via insulin receptor to begin a cascade of post-receptor events within the target cell. Phosphorylation stimulates insulin receptor substrates (IRS1-4) to promote glucose uptake through the transmembrane glucose transporter (GLUT4) and additionally intracellular protein synthesis. Tyrosine phosphorylation increments the tyrosine kinase activity of the insulin receptor, while serine phosphorylation inhibits it, and it appears that at least 50% of PCOS patients have excessive serine phosphorylation and inhibition of normal signaling (Tsilchorozidou, Overton et al. 2004). This influences merely glucose homeostasis and not the other pleiotropic activity of insulin, so that cell growth and protein synthesis continue. In addition, serine phosphorylation boosts activity of P450c17 in both the ovary and adrenal gland, hence promoting androgen synthesis, and this may be a reason for both insulin resistance and hyperandrogenism in some PCOS patients (Zhang, Rodriguez et al. 1995).

The source of hyperinsulinemia in patients with PCOS also remains unknown. The post receptor insulin signaling pathway and/or defective insulin secretion may be associated with an intrinsic abnormality (Holte, Bergh et al. 1995; Dunaif 1997). Probably, the metabolic abnormalities in PCOS begin very early in life, during the prenatal or prepubertal period, and an early exposure to androgens during growth may affect the body fat distribution and insulin action (Abbott, Dumesic et al. 2002; Eisner, Barnett et al. 2002). These observations have shown convincing proof that PCOS patients have insulin resistance and/or hyperinsulinemia, especially when they are anovulatory and obese with central fat distribution. Given that insulin resistance is an independent risk factor for metabolic abnormalities, the presence of insulin resistance in PCOS women implies the future possibility of cardiovascular disease and type 2 diabetes. Moreover, applying a cardiovascular risk score, insulin resistance in PCOS was established to be an important independent determining factor of cardiovascular risk in women with PCOS (Mather, Kwan et al. 2000).

The 2003 Rotterdam Consensus Conference (at least two of three features: oligo/anovulation, clinical and/or biochemical hyperandrogenism, polycystic ovaries) (2004) revised the 1990 US National Institutes of Health (NIH) definition of PCOS (hyperandrogenism and/or hyperandrogenemia plus oligo-ovulation, with the exclusion of other causes) (Zawadzki and Dunaif 1992), started a great debate. The majority of the studies investigating the metabolic associations of PCOS have used the 1990 NIH definition. Existing proofs support an increased risk of metabolic dysfunction in patients with clinical and/or biochemical hyperandrogenism and oligoovulation, and also in women with hyperandrogenism and normoovulation with polycystic ovaries (Azziz, Carmina et al. 2006). Women with or without oligoovulation with polycystic ovaries have nil or very subtle metabolic characteristics that makes it difficult for their involvement as a syndrome (Azziz, Carmina et al. 2006; Barber, Wass et al. 2007).

2.1.2 Dyslipidemia

Dyslipidemia is one of the most verified independent risk factors for the development of atherosclerotic cardiovascular disease, especially elevated low-density lipoprotein (LDL) and triglyceride (TG) levels. The most common metabolic abnormality in PCOS may be dyslipidemia, with a prevalence of up to 70% according to National Cholesterol Education Program criteria (Dunaif, Segal et al. 1989; Talbott, Clerici et al. 1998; Legro, Kunselman et al. 1999).

Insulin resistance, and its common, but not constant companion, compensatory hyperinsulinemia, have been linked with other different patterns of dyslipidemia. These include low levels of high-density lipoprotein(HDL)-cholesterol (HDL-C), increased values of triglycerides and total and low-density lipoprotein (LDL)-cholesterol (LDL-C), as well as varied LDL quality (Talbott, Clerici et al. 1998; Legro, Kunselman et al. 2001; Pirwany, Fleming et al. 2001; Essah, Nestler et al. 2008; Valkenburg, Steegers-Theunissen et al. 2008). However, lower HDL levels, higher low-density lipoprotein (LDL)/HDL ratios and higher triglyceride levels are seen most often in both lean and obese women with PCOS (Wild, Painter et al. 1985). This lipid pattern is similar to that found in T2DM. And it is mostly the result of IR that impairs the capability of insulin to suppress lipolysis, thereby expanding mobilization of free fatty acids from adipose stores. As a result, raised hepatic delivery of free fatty acids impairs insulin inhibition of hepatic very low-density lipoprotein 1 synthesis, causing altered catabolism of very low-density lipoprotein (Brunzell and Ayyobi 2003). Excessive adipose tissue increase insulin resistance, and this pattern is more common in obese patients with PCOS. These different patterns may be linked to the accompanying effects of IR and hyperandrogenism that merge with environmental (diet, physical exercise) and genetic factors (Dunaif 1997).

LDL subclasses are consequential predictors of CVD (Gardner, Fortmann et al. 1996). LDL particles are diverse in magnitude, density, and structure. CAD has been associated with small dense LDL particles and increased relative risk of CAD, that ranges from 3- to 7-fold (Austin, Breslow et al. 1988). Numerous studies have revealed a high prevalence of small LDL size in PCOS patients (Wild, Pierpoint et al. 2000; Dejager, Pichard et al. 2001). The differences in lipid profile are sharper at earlier ages and minor divergence is notable beyond the age of 40 years among to PCOS and control women, suggesting an incresaed risk for atherosclerosis at an earlier age (Talbott, Guzick et al. 1995; Talbott, Clerici et al. 1998). Existance of hormonal discordance may cause an earlier occurrence of atherosclerosis. Obesity and intraabdominal fat distribution in PCOS patients or may reflect the LDL-C increment with age among controls.

Recently, several studies have shown that similar changes of plasma lipids, distinct alterations of Lp and apoB substantially increase the cardiovascular risk (2002; Wierzbicki 2008). ApoB is the principal constitutional component of LDL and a true indicator of the number of particles promoting arteriosclerosis (2002). Some studies found no differences in apoB levels between women with PCOS and the controls (Valkenburg, Steegers-Theunissen et al. 2008). However, the others have shown significant increments in PCOS patients than the controls (Demirel, Bideci et al. 2007). Almost certainly, genetic and environmental influences may cause different lipid patterns. Based on these present data the determination of apoB levels is not advisable in women with PCOS.

Lipoprotein(a) is a miscellaneous class of lipoproteins constructed of an apo(a) molecule connected to an apoB-100 and a lipid. Lp(a) levels are determined genetically, and its metabolic characteristics are different from LDL. The concentration an Lp(a) is remaining stable during the life of a subject (Scanu 1992). Elevated Lp(a) concentrations represent an independent risk factor for cardiovascular events, associated to a raised risk of myocardium infarction, stroke and coronary heart disease (Sandkamp, Funke et al. 1990; Nagayama, Shinohara et al. 1994). Many studies and metaanalysis suggest that Lp(a) levels are increased in women with PCOS (Rizzo, Berneis et al. 2009; Toulis, Goulis et al. 2011).

Lipid disorders in PCOS appear to be connected to hyperinsulinemia (Mather, Kwan et al. 2000) and central obesity (Pirwany, Fleming et al. 2001). Some of the researchers suggested that androgen levels were associated with triglyceride levels, and lipids did not have any association (Legro, Kunselman et al. 2001). Nevertheless, others found no association between androgen levels and dyslipidemia (Pirwany, Fleming et al. 2001).

The current data suggest that distinct lipid profiles may be present in women with PCOS. Furthermore, distinctions among diverse racial and geographical characteristics cannot be entirely explained with body weight variations solely (Essah, Nestler et al. 2008; Valkenburg, Steegers-Theunissen et al. 2008). These distinctions may depend on the combination of genetic, environmental, and hormonal influences. In support of this issue, nonobese women with PCOS also can have raised levels of lipoprotein (a), a steady, genetically and racially determined, lipid-rich, LDL-like lipoprotein that is metabolically different from LDL-C (Scanu 1992; Rizzo, Berneis et al. 2009).

2.1.3 Hyperandrogenism

Hyperandrogenism is a dominant characteristic of PCOS with rises of ovarian androgens, testosterone, and androstenedione. Sex hormone binding globulin (SHBG) is usually low in PCOS, principally due to obesity, leading to higher free testosterone levels (Carmina 2002). Hyperandrogenism in PCOS patients, is an indefinite diagnosis of "androgen excess" that does not virilize. However, goes beyond the normal limits. Some depend on the clinical presentation of peripheral androgen excess in women, involving midline hirsutism, acne, and androgenic alopecia to make the diagnosis of hyperandrogenism as part of the PCOS phenotype (Hatch, Rosenfield et al. 1981; Lookingbill, Demers et al. 1991). Hirsutism is quite more common than the PCOS in the populations. Biochemical criteria, in contrast to clinical criteria, are more often used to report hyperandrogenism (Azziz, Ehrmann et al. 2001). Generally, it is concluded with serum tests to document increase in circulating androgen levels. In many multicenter clinical trials of women with PCOS, testosterone and/or some measurements of bioavailable testosterone has been frequently used to determine hyperandrogenism (Hines, Moran et al. 2001).

The gender distinction in vulnerability to cardiovascular disorder has been referred to the difference in sex steroids with oestrogen being seen as cardioprotective and androgens as a potential for exacerbating cardiovascular risk factors (Wu and von Eckardstein 2003). Clinical signs of hyperandrogenism, hirsutism and acne have been recognized as common characteristics of women suffering catheterization for coronary artery disease and were related with more serious disease (Wild, Grubb et al. 1990). There is little proof of an association among androgenic alopecia and raised cardiovascular risk in men, and there is even less in women (Rebora 2001). Iatrogenic hyperandrogenism in female-to-male transsexuals does not cause increased cardiovascular mortality (van Kesteren, Asscheman et al. 1997). Nevertheless, in an experimental model, testosterone management in female primates was related with raised premature atherogenesis, independent of lipid property (Adams, Williams et al. 1995). Equivalent trials in animal models of PCOS have not been reported to date.

The CVD is very low in premenopausal women and there was no evidence about correlation with increased androgens in circulation or urinary excretion with subsequently developed CVD (Gorgels, v d Graaf et al. 1997). Furthermore, prospective researches of postmenopausal populations, circulating androgen levels did not correlate with cardiovascular events (Price, Lee et al. 1997). The few studies that examined the correlation between endogenous androgens and the evolvement of cardiovascular disorder have not shown that androgen level performs a significant role in women with PCOS (Barrett-Connor and Goodman-Gruen 1995). The carotid intima-medial thickness (CIMT) has been shown to be inversely correlated with endogenous dehydroepiandrosterone sulphate (DHEAS) and testosterone in premenopausal and postmenopausal women (Bernini, Sgro et al. 1999).

It looks likely that in spite of the accepted consistent gender disproportion in the prevalence of cardiovascular disease, nonhormonal, genetic and environmental circumstances may play a greater role than that of androgens. In summary, the evidence for a association between hyperandrogenism per se and CVD in women is faint.

2.1.4 Novel risk factors

Recent cardiovascular studies have identified new biochemical markers for early atherosclerosis, and many of these have been found to be elevated in women with PCOS. Preliminary investigations suggest that serum biomarkers of cardiovascular disease, such as C-reactive protein (Kelly, Lyall et al. 2001; Mohlig, Spranger et al. 2004), adiponectin (Panidis, Kourtis et al. 2003; Spranger, Mohlig et al. 2004), plasminogen activator-1 (Sampson, Kong et al. 1996), endothelin-1 (Diamanti-Kandarakis, Spina et al. 2001), Von Willebrand factor (Dahlgren, Janson et al. 1994), homocysteine (Loverro, Lorusso et al. 2002) and markers of oxidative stress (Sabuncu, Vural et al. 2001) were abnormal in women with PCOS.

Whilst hyperhomocysteinemia is a risk factor for cardiovascular diseases, it has been assumed that homocysteine levels are higher in women with PCOS than controls. Homocysteine is an amino acid created by the transformation of methionine to cysteine. Homocysteine is metabolized by one of two mechanisms: trans-sulfuration and remethylation. This procedure needs vitamin B as a cofactor (Dahlgren, Janson et al. 1992; Talbott, Guzick et al. 1995; Wild, Pierpoint et al. 2000).

Potential pathophysiologic mechanisms of the impact of homocysteine comprise intensified peroxidation injury, proliferation of the smooth vessel, initiative of monocytic chemotaxis, enhanced cytotoxicity and inflammation, promotion of clotting, inhibition of anticoagulation, through effects on endothelial cells, and activation of platelet aggregation (Fermo, Vigano' D'Angelo et al. 1995; Mayer, Jacobsen et al. 1996; D'Angelo and Selhub 1997).

Numerous epidemiological reports have established hyperhomocysteinemia as an independent risk factor for cardiovascular disease, cerebrovascular disease, recurrent venous thromboembolism. It may arise from genetic defects in the enzymes within homocysteine pathways such as a methylene tetrahydrofolate reductase (MTHFR), imperfections in vitamin cofactors, or other causes, which contain drugs, such as fibrates and nicotinic acid and several chronic medical conditions (D'Angelo, Coppola et al. 2000; Orio, Palomba et al. 2003; Dierkes, Westphal et al. 2004; Baccarelli, Zanobetti et al. 2007). Many studies have evaluated homocysteine levels in women with PCOS. Most have revealed that women with PCOS have increased homocysteine levels when compared with controls (de la Calle, Gallardo et al. 2007; Atamer, Demir et al. 2008; Yilmaz, Pektas et al. 2008; Oktem, Ozcimen et al. 2009).

The role of inflammation in the evolvement of atherosclerosis has been well clarified. Epidemiological researches to have displayed that markers of inflammation, such as C-reactive protein (CRP) and white cell count, are independent predictors of cardiovascular disease odds. Several studies have been displayed elevated levels of high sensitivity CRP (Kelly, Lyall et al. 2001; Boulman, Levy et al. 2004), but not all (Mohlig, Spranger et al. 2004), in women with PCOS, independent of BMI. Recently, a higher white cell count was found to be correlated with a degree of insulin resistance in women with PCOS independent of BMI (Orio, Palomba et al. 2005). Predictors of vascular endothelial activation and damage, and oxidative stress has also been associated to a raised incidence of cardiovascular hazard, and peculiarities of these have been reported in women with PCOS. This issue is controversial if these correlations are independent of co-existent causes such as age, obesity, insulin resistance, blood pressure, serum glucose and lipid levels.

The circulating levels of tumour necrosis factor? α (TNF α), interleukin (IL)-6, as well as white blood count (WBC) and neutrophil count have been found to be elevated in PCOS patients compared with age- and /body mass index- (BMI-) matched controls (Alexander 1994; Kelly, Lyall et al. 2001; Amato, Conte et al. 2003). However, it has been revealed that obesity, and not PCOS status per se, was a major determinant of the circulating inflammatory markers TNF α, soluble type 2 TNF receptor, IL-6, and hs-CRP (Escobar-Morreale, Villuendas et al. 2003; Mohlig, Spranger et al. 2004). Increment in both low-grade chronic inflammation and insulin resistance in women with PCOS is related with raised central fat excess rather than PCOS status (Puder, Varga et al. 2005). Furthermore, TNF α is over expressed in adipose tissue and induces insulin resistance throughout acute and chronic effects on insulin-sensitive tissues (Hotamisligil, Shargill et al. 1993). The origin of redundant TNF α in PCOS is likely to be adipose tissue in the obese but remain obscure in lean women with PCOS. Nevertheless, increased visceral obesity could be a origin of redundant TNF α in lean women with PCOS. Other proinflammatory cytokine is IL-18, which was showed to be raised in PCOS patients (Stephens, Butts et al. 1992). IL-18 causes the production of TNF α which promotes the synthesis of IL-6, which is also thought about a strong risk marker for cardiovascular disease (Blankenberg, Tiret et al. 2002). Collectively, the above findings reveal that low-grade chronic inflammation could be a novel mechanism contributing to increased risk of coronary heart disease in PCOS.

Adiponectin, leptin and resistin, are bioactive peptides that are known as adipocyokines secreted by adipocytes, can affect insulin sensitivity and energy balance. Whether or not they have a function in the pathogenesis of PCOS is mysterious. Still the peculiarities in the plasma concentrations of adipocytokines independent of obesity and insulin resistance in PCOS have not been consistently demonstrated (Panidis, Kourtis et al. 2003; Spranger, Mohlig et al. 2004). The low plasma adiponectin levels have been related with an increased risk of the development of type 2 diabetes (Lindsay, Funahashi et al. 2002). Low adiponectin levels have also been connected with endothelial dysfunction (Tan, Xu et al. 2004), inflammation (Ouchi, Kihara et al. 2003) and coronary artery disease (Kumada, Kihara et al. 2003)

2.2 Clinical factors

2.2.1 Obesity

Obesity is a well defined independent risk factor for the development of type 2 diabetes and cardiovascular disorder. The western lifestyle is a major cause that increased the obesity prevalence (Kuczmarski, Flegal et al. 1994). The hyperinsulinemia appears to be the principal metabolic characteristic in normoglycemic normotensive obese subjects, while insulin resistance is not as extensive as formerly thought (Ferrannini, Natali et al. 1997). Most momentously, cardiovascular morbidity and mortality are raised in obese women independently of other hazardous influences (Manson, Colditz et al. 1990).

The PCOS patients are usually more obese than age matched controls, and have a rise of both BMI and waist/hip ratio (Talbott, Guzick et al. 1995). The appearance of obesity in women with PCOS diverges according to geographic location and the obese phenotype being remarkably common in the United States of America (Knochenhauer, Key et al. 1998). The UK researches showed the prevalence of obesity in PCO women was 35-38% (Kiddy, Sharp et al. 1990; Balen, Conway et al. 1995). The prevalance of PCOS was 10-38% in Mediterranean countries (Diamanti-Kandarakis, Kouli et al. 1999; Asuncion, Calvo et al. 2000) and Norman et al. found a prevalance as high as 63% in Australia (Norman, Masters et al. 1995).

Obesity is related with the insulin resistance, hypertension, dyslipidemia, subclinical inflammation and increased platelet activation, which are risk factors for atherosclerosis (Despres, Moorjani et al. 1990; Davi, Guagnano et al. 2002; Dalton, Cameron et al. 2003). A central obesity, which is demonstrated with an elevated waist/hip ratio, is an important and independent cardiovascular risk factor (Norman, Masters et al. 2001). The correlation between central obesity and cardiovascular disease in PCOS may be relatively linked to low plasma adiponectin levels, even though this postulate has not yet been seriously evaluated (Nishizawa, Shimomura et al. 2002).

2.2.2 Hypertension

Whether the prevalence of hypertension is increased in women with PCOS is obscure. Relevant researches to have utilized varying definitions of PCOS, and a wide diversity of techniques to evaluate blood pressure. Furthermore, studies, including those utilizing 24-h ambulatory blood pressure monitoring procedures, have stated inconsistent consequences (Dahlgren, Janson et al. 1992; Mather, Kwan et al. 2000; Wild, Pierpoint et al. 2000). Obese PCOS patients were found to have raised systolic but not diastolic BP compared to weight matched control women, although there was no divergence in blood pressure degrees between the non-obese group (Legro, Kunselman et al. 2001). Women with oligomenorrhea and hirsutism had increased levels of systolic and diastolic blood pressures compared to control women (Taponen, Martikainen et al. 2004). Additionally, some research indicated that an increased risk of having prehypertension (SBP 120 to 139 mm Hg or DBP 80 to 89 mmg Hg) in women with PCOS (Lo, Feigenbaum et al. 2006), a condition related with a two-times an increased risk of death from a cardiovascular disease (Masi, Feigenbaum et al. 1995).

However, existing data need to be assessed with caution, since small differences in blood pressure could have a great effect on the population cardiovascular risk (Rose 1981). The absence of momentous association with hypertension is surprising while considering the close link between PCOS and the metabolic syndrome. Pertinent studies have, however, utilized variable definitions of PCOS and employed a wide variety of techniques to assess blood pressure.

2.2.3 Metabolic syndrome

Metabolic syndrome, or the insulin resistance syndrome which has been known as a constellation of endocrine and biochemical markers that places affected individuals at important cardiovascular risk. The metabolic syndrome is described by the presence of three out of the five following criteria: fasting serum glucose of 100 mg/dL or greater, blood pressure higher than 130/85 mmHg, fasting triglyceride level greater than 150 mg/dL; serum high density lipoprotein cholesterol less than 50 mg/dL in females and a woman's waist circumference equal to or greater than 35 inches (88 cm) (2002).

Individuals with the metabolic syndrome have a raised likelihood of having CVD and increased all-cause mortality, nevertheless, in the absence of diabetes or cardiovascular disease at baseline (Korytkowski, Mokan et al. 1995). PCOS patients have been found to have an increased incidence of the metabolic syndrome (Dahlgren, Landin et al. 1998; Baillargeon, Jakubowicz et al. 2004). The prevalence has been stated to be as high as 43% in these patients, which is twofold more than the age-adjusted prevalence rate of 24% nationally, displayed in the NHANES III survey data analysis (Morin-Papunen, Vauhkonen et al. 2000). Dokras et al. revealed the age- and BMI-adjusted prevalence of the metabolic syndrome to be 47% in women with PCOS compare to 4.3% in controls, which renders to an eleven-fold increased risk (Elter, Imir et al. 2002).

A waist circumference >88 cm (35 in) or >85 cm defined a central obesity, as proposed by the International Diabetes Foundation, appears to be the most common element of the metabolic syndrome in PCOS. Unexpectedly, Dokras et al. also displayed a 23% prevalence of the metabolic syndrome in those women with PCOS under 30 years of age, compared to 0% for their counterparts without PCOS and 6.7% prevalence among the same demografic values in women in the NHANES study (Elter, Imir et al. 2002; Shroff, Kerchner et al. 2007). Consequently, these researchers suggested that all women with PCOS be screened for the metabolic syndrome. Other experts related to this area also agreed with this suggestion.

Furthermore, the important issue is that the usefulness of the metabolic syndrome as a predictor of cardiovascular disease and type 2 diabetes was recently elucidated when compared with established alternative, more specific risk prediction models. The Diabetes Predicting Model and the Framingham cardiovascular risk score estimate the future risk of developing type 2 diabetes and cardiovascular disease respectively. They take into consideration several risk factors such as ethnicity, age, gender, fasting blood glucose, blood pressure, lipids, smoking status and family history. When compared with the metabolic syndrome in a population-based cohort study these specific prediction models were found to have raised the sensitivity and specificity in predicting diabetes and cardiovascular disease respectively (Stern, Williams et al. 2004).

2.2.4 Mood disturbances and reduced quality of life

Accumulating data indicated that mood disturbances, principally severe depression were independent risk factors for CVD (Ounpuu, Negassa et al. 2001) and prevalent in PCOS (Jones, Hall et al. 2008; Bishop, Basch et al. 2009). Various studies displayed increased prevalence of depression and anxiety in women with PCOS. These mood alterations and impaired quality of life cause tiredness, sleep disturbances, phobia, appetite changes, and binge eating (Hollinrake, Abreu et al. 2007; Bishop, Basch et al. 2009; Jedel, Waern et al. 2010). Consequenctly, depressed women with PCOS have higher BMI and greater IR as CVD risk factors than nondepressed women with PCOS without discrepancies in androgen status(Hollinrake, Abreu et al. 2007), whereas weight loss by an energy-restricted diet ameliorates their depression and quality of life (Thomson, Buckley et al. 2010). It remains to be resolved how mood disturbances as CVD risk factors are associated with shifted stress responsiveness in PCOS patients, as demonstrated by excessive ACTH and cortisol stress responses, disabled IL-6 reply following stres (Benson, Arck et al. 2009), and raised sympathetic nerve activity (Sverrisdottir, Mogren et al. 2008).

2.2.5 Obstructive sleep apnea

Reports in recent years have revealed on another comorbidity connected with PCOS, obstructive sleep apnea (OSA). OSA has significant clinical consequences, involving raised daytime sleepiness, decreased quality of life, and lessened cognitive performance. Serious cardiovascular effects have also been shown to consequences from OSA, comprising hypertension (Brooks, Horner et al. 1997; Lavie, Herer et al. 2000),stroke (Dyken, Somers et al. 1996), and myocardial infarction (Hung, Whitford et al. 1990). Fogel et al. was shown that obese women with PCOS had substantially raised Apnea- Hypopnea Index (AHI) when compared to age- and weight-matched controls. Moreover, this research demonstrated that PCOS patients were also nine times as more likely to suffer from OSA when compared to the control group (Fogel, Malhotra et al. 2001). Another study performed by Vgontzas et al. displayed sleep-disturbed breathing prevalence 30 times more in PCOS patients than the control group (Vgontzas, Legro et al. 2001).

The high prevalence of OSA has been regard to be a role of both increased levels of testosterone as well as the obesity that prevalently accompanies PCOS. Nevertheless, it looks that the high commonness of OSA in PCOS cannot be completely explained for based on these two causes solely (Nitsche and Ehrmann 2010). Insulin resistance was found to be a sharper predictor of sleep disordered breathing than was age, circulating testosterone concentrations and BMI (Vgontzas, Legro et al. 2001). It also revealed that women with PCOS taking oral contraceptives were reduced probability to have sleep disordered breathing, uniform with new consequences from the Sleep Heart Health Study Research Group in which hormone-replacement treatment was related with an inferior possibility of sleep disordered breathing among post-menopausal women (Shahar, Redline et al. 2003).

Obese PCOS patients are more likely to suffer from OSA compared to lean patients. The important morbidity and mortality, associated with this condition. PCOS patients should be screened meticulously with regard to characteristics of daytime sleepiness, morning headaches, snoring, and other symptoms of OSA and directed for proper studies to verify this diagnosis.

3. Subclinical atherosclerosis

Even though the epidemiologic data on cardiovascular events are sparse in women with PCOS, the evaluation of cardiovascular structure and function is providing proof that PCOS and its related clinical phenotype clearly affects the arterial wall and/or myocardium.

3.1 Carotid intima media thickness

The CIMT has been displayed in numerous studies to predict cardiovascular events, with increasing CIMT correlated with an elevated age-adjusted cardiovascular risk (Bots, Dijk et al. 2002). Increased carotid intima media thickness (IMT), reminiscent of a raised risk for atherosclerosis, was displayed in a small group of PCOS patients over 40 years of age. However, there were no important discrepancies in the prevalence of carotid plaque amongst cases and controls (Guzick, Talbott et al. 1996). This result was independent of dyslipidemia but not plasma insulin levels and obesity. Nevertheless, Talbott et al. stated that CIMT measurements were only distinctive in older PCOS patients compared with controls, and after adjusting for coexistent cardiovascular risk factors PCOS was not a significant predictor of CIMT. This study additionally reported a substantially greater carotid plaque index in the PCOS subjects compared with controls. These results imply that in women with PCOS, subclinical atherosclerosis may not be obvious up to the time of the perimenopause (Talbott, Guzick et al. 2000).

Recently, two researches to have displayed a significant difference in CIMT among young, normal weight PCOS patients compared with controls (Orio, Palomba et al. 2004; Vural, Caliskan et al. 2005). Vural et al. demonstrated that PCOS, BMI and a reduced sex hormone binding globulin were all independent predictors of CIMT (Vural, Caliskan et al. 2005). However, the report by Orio et al ., showed a strong association between CIMT and the free androgen index that suggests a contribution of hyperandrogenemia to evolvement of atherosclerosis in PCOS (Orio, Palomba et al. 2004). Contrarily, in a larger study raised CIMT was conversely correlated with plasma DHEAS and androstenedione concentrations, proposing a fascinating vasculoprotective influence of hyperandrogenemia in PCOS (Vryonidou, Papatheodorou et al. 2005). Meyer et al. also found a similar vasculoprotective effect of DHEAS in a study involving 80 obese women with PCOS, where higher DHEAS corresponded to notably lower CIMT (Meyer, McGrath et al. 2005). Whether the DHEAS has actually beneficial effects on atherogenesis in PCOS obscure and needs further studies to elucidate this issue.

3.2 Coronary artery calcification

Coronary artery calcification (CAC) demonstrates the grade of atherosclerosis and is early marker for clinical events. The electron beam computer tomography, has been employed to show raised arterial calcification in the coronary circulation in PCOS women compared with controls (Christian, Dumesic et al. 2003). Since adjusting for BMI, dyslipidemia remained a useful prognosticator of coronary calcification. The research of Mayo Clinic found a 3-fold rise in CAC in non-diabetic PCOS cases than population controls (Christian, Dumesic et al. 2003). Moreover, when these same participants were compared to obese control women, the participants with PCOS had 2-fold higher degrees of CAC. The intriguing prospective, case-control research with over a nine year follow-up period in PCOS reported by Talbott et al. display an increased incidence of coronary and aortic arterial calcification (Talbott, Zborowski et al. 2004). Young obese PCOS patients have been shown to have a five times raised prevalence of subclinical CAD with the presence of momentous CAC as contrasted to age- and weight matched women (Shroff, Kerchner et al. 2007). The features of metabolic syndrome affect the grade of calcification, comprising central obesity, elevated blood pressure and dyslipidemia, and as a consequence insulin resistance. In that study, the degree of aortic calcification was also positively associated with plasma testosterone concentrations, questioning a presumed atheroprotective nature of hyperandrogenemia in PCOS. These reports, accompanied with angiographic statistics in women displayed a correlation among coronary artery disease and polycystic ovaries (Birdsall, Farquhar et al. 1997).

3.3 Endothelial dysfunction

Endothelial dysfunction is recognized to be an early characteristic in the progression of atherosclerosis, and the greater part of researches of macro- and micro-vascular endothelial function in women with PCOS has displayed significant peculiarities. The findings of the studies revealed that arterial dilatory function was a sign for the presence of endothelial dysfunction in distinct arterial beds in women with PCOS and was related to endothelial dysfunction among insulin resistance and less consistently to hyperandrogenemia. Related mechanisms almost certainly account for the effect of insulin resistance on the biology of NO in both conduit and resistance arteries in PCOS patients (Paradisi, Steinberg et al. 2001; Kelly, Speirs et al. 2002; Orio, Palomba et al. 2004). These studies collectively confirmed that increased arterial stiffness, myocardial and endothelial dysfunction showed solid pathophysiological proof for arterial atherosclerosis in women with PCOS. Many of these studies have shown a correlation between insulin resistance and cardiovascular abnormalities, and supported the hypothesis that insulin resistance remains at the vascular level in women with PCOS. However, still needs further proof for the associate with the clinical cardiovascular events.

3.4 Ventricular function

One of the early manifestations of diabetic cardiomyopathy is left ventricular (LV) diastolic dysfunction which has been recognized as a predictor for cardiovascular events in hypertensive patients (Schannwell, Schneppenheim et al. 2002; Schillaci, Pasqualini et al. 2002). Its etiology is multifactorial and refers to hypertension, coronary artery disease, insulin resistance, autonomic neuropathy, microangiopathy, dyslipidemia, endothelial dysfunction and oxidative stres (Brutsaert, Sys et al. 1993). The case control prospective studies that utilize echocardiographic methods demonsrated that women with PCOS were found to have a raised isovolumetric relaxation time (IVRT), an indicator of the early LV diastolic dysfunction, and lower ejection fraction in contrast to weight matched controls. In addition, an important clear connection among plasma insulin levels and IVRT was displayed in PCOS patients (Tiras, Yalcin et al. 1999). These results were consistent with another study which demonstrated an independent association between hyperinsulinemia and LV mass (Orio, Palomba et al. 2004).

The postulate that insulin resistance may contribute to myocardial dysfunction in PCOS has been supported with these studies' findings.

3.5 Aortic stiffness

The peripheral circulation arterial stiffness is related to raised systolic blood pressure, pulse pressure and ventricular load, as well as to decreased diastolic perfusion of the coronary blood flow. Arterial stiffness may be assessed by two approaches. One is the ultrasonographic evaluation of carotid artery distensibility by measuring pulse wave velocity (PWV) and the other one analysis of the diastolic part of the radial waveform (Bots, Dijk et al. 2002). Arterial stiffness is increased in other diseases such as in renal failure it has been indicated to have prognostic value for cardiovascular events (London, Marchais et al. 2004). Kelly et al. found increased pulse wave velocity of the brachial artery, but not of the aorta, in PCOS patients in a small case control study (Kelly, Speirs et al. 2002). Likewise, Lakhani et al. showed raised stiffness of both internal and external carotid arteries in women with both PCOS and PCO (ultrasonographic polycystic ovaries alone) compared with controls. Multivariate analysis implied independent influences of PCOS and PCO on arterial stiffness (Lakhani, Constantinovici et al. 2000).

4. Cardiovascular events

In spite of the fact that cardiovascular risk factors are more frequently found in PCOS patients, reliable proof for a raised prevalence of cardiovascular disease is lacking. The predicted relative risk of myocardial infarction was found 7,4 by the calculated risk factor profile in a small group of women (n = 33) with histopathological verification of polycystic ovaries (PCO) compared with aged-matched controls (Dahlgren, Janson et al. 1992).

A subsequent study that included 142 women undergoing coronary angiography revealed that polycystic ovaries were independently correlated with the presence of an extent of coronary atherosclerosis determined during catheterization. The examination of pelvic ultrasonography imaging showed that forty two percent of these women had polycystic ovaries. Moreover, these patients had more extensive coronary artery disease than the group without polycystic ovaries, established on a number of segments by more than 50% stenosis (Fogel, Malhotra et al. 2001).

Nevertheless, a larger retrospective cohort found that PCOS patients (n = 345) diagnosed primarily with ovarian morphology, had further cardiovascular risk factors, comprising obesity, diabetes, hypertension and hyperlipidemia. Their mortality and morbidity from coronary heart disease didn't show a disparity from age-matched controls (n = 1060) (Wild, Pierpoint et al. 2000). This remarkable result could be explained with the ascertainment bias, to application of a non-standard description of PCOS, or perhaps to a cardiovascular defensive impact of hyperandrogenemia. Even though, after adjusting for BMI, the odd's ratios for developing diabetes and cerebrovascular disease in this analysis were raised considerably at 2.3 and 2.8, respectively.

The Women's Ischemia Syndrome Evaluation (WISE) is the most important study that evaluated both cardiovascular risk and consequences in women with PCOS. WISE is a multicenter research that intends to ameliorate diagnostic testing for ischemic heart disease in women and to study pathophysiology and prognosis in women with symptoms and proof of myocardial ischemia in the absence or presence of obstructive coronary artery disease (CAD). The researchers included 390 postmenopausal women and diagnosed PCOS with the rise in blood serum androgen concentrations integrated with a premenopausal history of irregular menses (n =104). Notably, the prevalence (27%) of PCOS was considerably higher than the population anticipation (5%–8%). However, women with ischemia may represent a refined pool for women with PCOS. Clinically most significant consequence is the cumulative 5-year cardiovascular event-free survival was 78.9% for 104 women with PCOS and 88.7% for 286 women without PCOS (Shaw, Bairey Merz et al. 2008).

Two more studies provided further support to the link between PCOS and CVD. One of them is a cross-sectional study, which included 713 postmenopausal women (mean age, 73.8 yr) and found in nondiabetic women with intact ovaries, a step-by-step categorized association between CVD and quantities of features of assumed PCOS, as described by premenopausal menstrual irregularity, hirsutism, or present biochemical hyperandrogenism (Krentz, von Muhlen et al. 2007). The other case-control study recruited 414 postmenopausal women (mean age, 60.4 yr), used premenopausal menstrual irregularity as a putative sign of PCOS, and found an increased odd's ratio for coronary vascular disorder (Azevedo, Duarte et al. 2006).

Since the majority of studies centered on surrogate results and there are weak at detecting true discrepancies in these consequences, we need extended-course of data to evaluate real risk.

5. Management of CVD risk factors

The PCOS treatment aims at amelioration of ovarian function, involving regulating and averting anovulatory uterine hemorrhagia, diminishing obesity, controlling cardiovascular risk factors such as insulin resistance, diabetes, hypertension, hyperlipidemia. Nevertheless, there is no better treatment alternative distinct from lifestyle modification. Numerous researches indicated that improving insulin sensitivity with lifestyle modifications or pharmacological treatment can diminish circulating androgen levels, and increase spontaneous ovulation and pregnancy.

5.1 Lifestyle modification

The most valuable approaches for improving insulin sensitivity in overweight, obese PCOS patients are diet, weight reduction, and physical activity. Obesity has changed into an epidemic in most parts of the world and has a marked on reproductive and metabolic peculiarities in women with PCOS. Regrettably there are no optimized medical therapies at this point that causes a permanent weight loss. Moreover, it was reported that 90-95% of subjects who achieved a weight loss will generally relapse (Rosenbaum, Leibel et al. 1997). The efficacious surgical alternative for the morbidly obese PCOS patients may be a bariatric surgery. However, there has been a few reports of this intervention in this special group.

The lifestyle modification for overweight/ obese patients, comprising diet, exercise, termination of smoking, and behavioral modification (Norman, Davies et al. 2002), may have beneficial effects to decrease CVD risk (De Backer, Ambrosioni et al. 2003). The researches revealed that short-period weight-loss intervention in PCOS patients lowers abdominal fat (Andersen, Seljeflot et al. 1995; Holte, Bergh et al. 1995), lessens androgen levels (Holte, Bergh et al. 1995), IR and in addition ameliorates dyslipidemia, depression, and quality of life, even though long-term weight loss is improbable (Andersen, Seljeflot et al. 1995; Thomson, Buckley et al. 2010).

Numerous studies in PCOS patients have demonstrated, that weight reduction can ameliorate the main characteristics of the endocrine syndrome of PCOS. Weight reduction decrease circulating androgen levels and restart the menstrual cycle (Guzick, Wing et al. 1994; Okajima, Koyanagi et al. 1994; Clark, Ledger et al. 1995).These alterations can be obtained with a weight loss as small as 5% of the initial weight (Franks, Kiddy et al. 1991; Kiddy, Hamilton-Fairley et al. 1992). Additional advantages that have been reported to have lowered circulating insulin levels (Kiddy, Hamilton-Fairley et al. 1989; Kiddy, Hamilton-Fairley et al. 1992). The reduction of free testosterone concentrations, subsequent weight loss mostly mediated through increases by SHBG (Franks, Kiddy et al. 1991; Kiddy, Hamilton-Fairley et al. 1992).

The hypocaloric, low saturated fat, increased mono- and polyunsaturated fat nutrition is advocated, simultaneously with at least 30 min of intermediate-strength physical activity every day to maintain weight. Together both decrease BMI and ameliorate IR and cardiopulmonary function in overweight/obese PCOS patients (Vigorito, Giallauria et al. 2007) and performed greater decreases in fat mass in PCOS women (Bruner, Chad et al. 2006). Altering a dietary macronutrient constitution does not offer a benefit for weight loss over prevalent dietetic approaches solely (Moran, Pasquali et al. 2009).

However, the majority of PCOS patients difficult to achieve desirable weight loss, despite a caloric reduction and modification to healthier diets and physical activity. It may be even harder for these subjects to maintain weight loss, especially whether they are insulin resistant. As well as 10-30% of women with PCOS are lean, weight loss is not a choice for their management.

5.2 Insulin sensitizers

Medications developed to treat type 2 diabetes that have insulin sensitizing properties (ie, metformin and thiazolidinediones) have been utilized to treat PCOS, because both diseases are thought to be developed based on impaired insulin action. This class of medication enhance insulin sensitivity and transform impaired to normal glucose tolerance in non-diabetic women with PCOS. These drugs, additionally improve metabolic predictors of cardiovascular risk in PCOS patients, comprising serum triglycerides, PAI-I, and lower blood pressure (Diamanti-Kandarakis, Kouli et al. 1998; Moghetti, Castello et al. 2000). The data provided from the UKPDS, a research of diabetic men and women, showed that there may be lesser cardiovascular events in insulin-resistant individuals treated with insulin-sensitizing drugs (1998).

5.2.1 Metformin

Metformin is one of the most frequently prescribed drugs to treat PCOS. Metformin has constantly shown an insulin lowering effect, and that may be its prime mechanism of action. Metformin was certified for the usage of type 2 diabetes by the FDA in 1994, although has been used clinically for approximately to 20 years formerly in other parts of the world (Coetzee and Jackson 1979).

Study results regarding the effects of metformin on primary prevention of CVD are not coherent (Moghetti, Castello et al. 2000; Diamanti-Kandarakis, Alexandraki et al. 2005; Rautio, Tapanainen et al. 2005). Metformin has a little influence on body weight (less than 2-3% of BMI) (Moghetti, Castello et al. 2000; Rautio, Tapanainen et al. 2005; Nieuwenhuis-Ruifrok, Kuchenbecker et al. 2009) and may ameliorate atherogenic dyslipidemia, raising HDL-C and lowering triglycerides (Rautio, Tapanainen et al. 2005; Trolle, Flyvbjerg et al. 2007). Nevertheless, no alterations in HDL-C or triglycerides were seen in some studies (Banaszewska, Pawelczyk et al. 2009). Metformin cannot improve LDL-C or non-HDL-C (Rautio, Tapanainen et al. 2005; Trolle, Flyvbjerg et al. 2007; Banaszewska, Pawelczyk et al. 2009). Furthermore, several studies with metformin have shown that, it lessens of circulating C-reactive protein, PAI-1 (Velazquez, Acosta et al. 1997; Morin-Papunen, Rautio et al. 2003) and may ameliorate premature atherosclerosis, decrease carotid IMT and enhance endothelial function (Diamanti-Kandarakis, Alexandraki et al. 2005; Agarwal, Rice et al. 2010).

The research of Sharma et al. investigated the efficacy of metformin in averting progression to type 2 diabetes, particularly in PCOS patients. During 43.3 months of treatment with metformin, 5% (N.=2) of the 39 patients with normal glucose tolerance at baseline transformed to impaired glucose tolerance, bearing an annual conversion rate of 1.4%. The published article's stated a 16-19% annual conversion rate for PCOS women, therefore, rendering a 11-fold decrease in the annual conversion to impaired glucose tolerance in this metformin given PCOS women. Moreover, none of the fifty PCOS women developed diabetes throughout the study period (Sharma, Wickham et al. 2007).

5.2.2 Thiazolidinediones

Thiazolidinediones (TZDs) have been proposed as a treatment option for many of the metabolic aspects of PCOS. These drugs act by increasing insulin stimulated glucose uptake, principally in adipose and skeletal muscle tissues. The activation of γ-peroxisome proliferation activator receptors (PPAR-γ) activates the genes that encode insulin. Troglitazone was the first to be used in this class. Troglitazone treatment improved endothelial function in obese PCOS patients when compared to age and weight matched controls (Paradisi, Steinberg et al. 2003) . The same result was obtained with rosiglitazone (Tarkun, Cetinarslan et al. 2005) and pioglitazone (Romualdi, Guido et al. 2003). Troglitazone additionally lowered circulating insulin levels, improved hirsutism, and increased the ovulation rates of PCOS patients (Paradisi, Steinberg et al. 2003)(Dunaif, Scott et al. 1996). A study examined the effects of metformin, rosiglitazone, and a combination of these drugs in non-obese PCOS patients with no clinical or biochemical proof of insulin resistance. Together with other findings, measures of insulin sensitivity was ameliorated meaningfully with metformin and combination therapy, but not with rosiglitazone solely (Baillargeon, Jakubowicz et al. 2004).

Troglitazone and rosiglitazone, at present, are not available due to liver toxicity and cardiovascular side effects respectively. Pioglitazone is the only available molecule in this class and to date did not have the hepatic side effects of their predecessors. A new study closely assessed cardiovascular risk factors in women with PCOS randomized to pioglitazone or placebo for 16 weeks (Glintborg, Hojlund et al. 2008). Enhancement of insulin sensitivity determined with clamp technique, however a serum marker of atherosclerosis sCD36 and hs-CRP significantly diminished. Insignificant alterations were measured in body weight or body composition in the treatment patients, which was unexpected, given the tendency to weight gain with thiazolidinedione remedies. Another recent analysis randomized 60 women with PCOS for 24 weeks to exenatide (a glucagon-like peptide-1 [GLP-1] analogue in the incretin class of drugs), metformin, or a combination of both (Elkind-Hirsch, Marrioneaux et al. 2008). The research revealed greater weight loss with exenatide than with metformin and found an additive effect of both. Even though no serious side effects (ie, pancreatitis with exenatide) were noted althought the knowledge with incretins in women with PCOS is very limited.

5.3 Cholesterol lowering drugs

The HMG-CoA reductase inhibitors are a class of cholesterol- lowering agents, also recognized as statins, are blocking the rate limiting step of cholesterol synthesis. Restriction of mevalonate production may furthermore cause diminished maturation of insulin receptors, inhibition of steroidogenesis (via restricting the substrate cholesterol), and change of signal transduction pathways that mediate cellular proliferation (Kodaman and Duleba 2008). They are thought to have a favorable influence on cardiovascular risk independent of their lipid-lowering effect as well, expectedly by pleiotropic activity on systemic inflammation and oxidative stress, the mechanism of which is still to be determined. Stress and inflammation are also thought to play a role in the progression of ovarian theca cell hyperplasia, lead to anovulation and hyperandrogenism in PCOS.

Even though several lipid-lowering medications have been tried (Rizzo, Berneis et al. 2008; Rosenzweig, Ferrannini et al. 2008), only statins have been adequately studied in women with PCOS and have efficiently lowered LDL-C levels (Banaszewska, Pawelczyk et al. 2009; Sathyapalan, Kilpatrick et al. 2009) . Several studies found that, statins decrease IR and inflammation, reduce serum total and free testosterone concentrations, and ameliorate endothelial dysfunction in PCOS patients (Duleba, Banaszewska et al. 2006; Banaszewska, Pawelczyk et al. 2009; Sathyapalan, Kilpatrick et al. 2009). Nevertheless, their usage in gestation is contraindicated, and contraception is needed.

Patients with serious dyslipidemia that is not adequately corrected by lifestyle modification and statins may need double pharmacotherapy. It has been found that the addition of metformin does not ameliorate lipid levels furthermore (Banaszewska, Pawelczyk et al. 2009). Statins combined with a fibrate may be required when hypertriglyceridemia and low HDL levels coexist. Fenofibrate is favored because of less drug interactions and the diminished possibility of myopathy (Zambon and Cusi 2007; Rosenzweig, Ferrannini et al. 2008). Nicotinic acid causes a beneficial effect on lipoproteins however needs cautious monitoring for deterioration of glycemic control (Rosenzweig, Ferrannini et al. 2008).

5.4 Hypertension theraphy

Antihypertensive drug medication is recommended for blood pressure of more than 140 mmHg systolic or 90 mmHg diastolic. Since milder elevation of BP (or prehypertension), increase CVD risk, diminishing BP to 120/80 mm Hg is desirable for longtime CVD protection (Rosenzweig, Ferrannini et al. 2008). Most of the researchers recommend merging pharmacotherapy accompanied by lifestyle modification for incessant hypertension in PCOS patients. Even though some investigators favor angiotensin-converting enzyme inhibitors and angiotensin receptor blockers over diuretics and beta-blockers, utilitization of angiotensin-converting enzyme inhibitors, angiotensin receptor blockers, diuretics and beta-blockers is contraindicated in pregnancy and requires contraception.

5.5 Antiobesity medications

Phenteramine, sibutramine, and orlistat are FDA-approved weight loss medicines. A number of researches have found that sibutramine combined with a hypocaloric diet enhances weight loss, improves IR, and hypertriglyceridemia, decrease serum free testosterone concentrations, to a greater extent than hypocaloric diet alone. However, this drug may raise diastolic BP and heart rate and is not approved in the course of gestation. Orlistat causes a smaller degree of weight loss. Since the clinical experience with these agents is limited in PCOS and unexpected side effects may happen, authorities do not advocate the utilitization of weight loss medicines in women with PCOS.

6. Conclusion and future aspects

Although the epidemiologic data is uncertain, current study results strongly support a correlation between PCOS and cardiovascular risk factors, which are represented in Figure 1. Discrepancies among some of the reports reviewed in this chapter, may be due to small sample sizes, bias in case-control designs and the non-standard delineations of PCOS criteria.

Data accumulated to date, indicate that insulin resistance, and obesity may be responsible for early ventricular functional abnormalities, arterial stiffness, endothelial dysfunction and both carotid and coronary atherosclerosis. These abnormalities may be detrimental consequences of insulin resistance per se, such as dyslipoproteinemia, hypertension, low grade inflammation, raised oxidative stress, changed hemostasis and coagulation system alterations. The diminished synthesis of nitric oxide (NO) and excess production of peroxinitrite are apparently principal factors to initiate endothelial dysfunction and atherothrombosis.

The function of hyperandrogenemia in subscribing to the cardiovascular abnormalities surveyed remains obscure and debatable. Most researches detected androgens as a cardiovascular risk in women with PCOS. Even though the minority of reports examined indicated an independent correlation of androgens with impaired cardiovascular structure or function. This additionally strengthens the thought that cardiovascular risk in PCOS resides to insulin resistance rather than hyperandrogenemia. Furthermore, some studies showed that in PCOS patients, androgens, particularly DHEAS, have been a negative association with CIMT.

Weight loss is realizable with lifestyle alterations, bariatric surgery, and pharmaceutical treatment, involving antiobesity and antidiabetic medications. Insulin sensitizers and statins, particularly in combination with hormonal remedies such as OCPs, oral contraceptives seem to have beneficial properties. Nonetheless, greater and longer trials are required previously to elucidate, which is the best treatment to impede cardiovascular events in women with PCOS can be advocated.

The postulation for the development of cardiovascular disease in PCOS founded on the studies surveyed and permitting the illustration in Figure 1.It summarizes possible pathways throughout the cardiovascular risk factors to CVD. However, the presence of these cardiovascular risk factors in women with PCOS, at this time sufficient prospective results that supporting the actual prevalence of cardiovascular events in PCOS patiens are lacking.

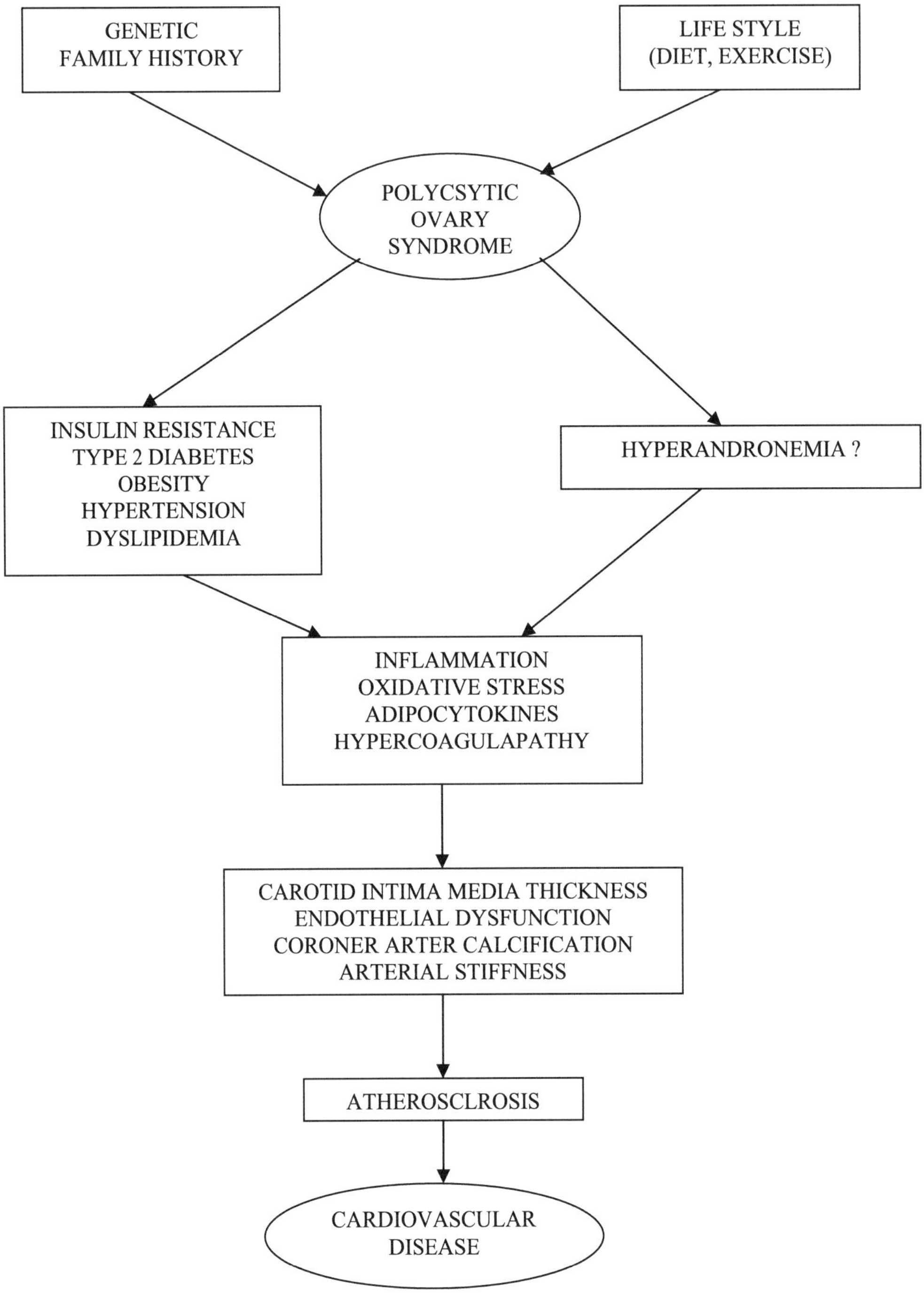

Fig. 1. Postulation for the pathogenesis of cardiovascular disease in PCOS. This figure outlines possible pathways which cardiovascular risk factors associated with PCOS may render into manifest cardiovascular disease.

Definitive prospective data to support a rise in adverse cardiovascular events in women with PCOS is non-existent. However, the most recent studies have firmed up the connection among women with PCOS and CVD events, even though they tend to present in menopause and not in reproductive-age women. Former prediction models have appraised a proportional risk of myocardial infarction of 7.4 PCOS patients. Nevertheless, a large retrospective report of PCOS women showed elevated ratios of diabetes and cerebrovascular disease but not cardiovascular disease, proposing that the earlier estimate of cardiovascular risk may have been extreme. Consequently, that researches perform hereafter have to analyses cardiovascular health results and endeavour to clarify those subgroups that are sharper risk for cardiovascular disease in women with PCOS.

From a clinical aspect, the current statistics imply that management should focus on the designation and treatment of peculiar cardiovascular risk factors recognized to occur more frequently PCOS patients. In particular, lifestyle modification, the avoidance of weight gain and obesity, and the long-term surveillance for evolvement of type 2 diabetes should be accented. After menopause conventional cardiovascular risk accelerates in women, have to be evaluated with precisely mentioning to PCOS. The consequences of interferences such as exogenous oestrogens and anti-androgen treatment on cardiovascular risk in PCOS also required to be investigated further. The high prevalence of this disease in reproductive age women, and the possible correlation with cardiovascular disease, cause future examinations in this issue a priority importance from both a public health and clinical aspect.

7. References

(1998). "Effect of intensive blood-glucose control with metformin on complications in overweight patients with type 2 diabetes (UKPDS 34). UK Prospective Diabetes Study (UKPDS) Group." Lancet 352(9131): 854-865.

(2002). "Third Report of the National Cholesterol Education Program (NCEP) Expert Panel on Detection, Evaluation, and Treatment of High Blood Cholesterol in Adults (Adult Treatment Panel III) final report." Circulation 106(25): 3143-3421.

(2004). "Revised 2003 consensus on diagnostic criteria and long-term health risks related to polycystic ovary syndrome (PCOS)." Hum Reprod 19(1): 41-47.

Abbott, D. H., D. A. Dumesic, et al. (2002). "Developmental origin of polycystic ovary syndrome - a hypothesis." J Endocrinol 174(1): 1-5.

Adams, M. R., J. K. Williams, et al. (1995). "Effects of androgens on coronary artery atherosclerosis and atherosclerosis-related impairment of vascular responsiveness." Arterioscler Thromb Vasc Biol 15(5): 562-570.

Agarwal, N., S. P. Rice, et al. (2010). "Metformin reduces arterial stiffness and improves endothelial function in young women with polycystic ovary syndrome: a randomized, placebo-controlled, crossover trial." J Clin Endocrinol Metab 95(2): 722-730.

Alexander, R. W. (1994). "Inflammation and coronary artery disease." N Engl J Med 331(7): 468-469.

Amato, G., M. Conte, et al. (2003). "Serum and follicular fluid cytokines in polycystic ovary syndrome during stimulated cycles." Obstet Gynecol 101(6): 1177-1182.

Andersen, P., I. Seljeflot, et al. (1995). "Increased insulin sensitivity and fibrinolytic capacity after dietary intervention in obese women with polycystic ovary syndrome." Metabolism 44(5): 611-616.

Asuncion, M., R. M. Calvo, et al. (2000). "A prospective study of the prevalence of the polycystic ovary syndrome in unselected Caucasian women from Spain." J Clin Endocrinol Metab 85(7): 2434-2438.

Atamer, A., B. Demir, et al. (2008). "Serum levels of leptin and homocysteine in women with polycystic ovary syndrome and its relationship to endocrine, clinical and metabolic parameters." J Int Med Res 36(1): 96-105.

Azevedo, G. D., J. M. Duarte, et al. (2006). "[Menstrual cycle irregularity as a marker of cardiovascular risk factors at postmenopausal years]." Arq Bras Endocrinol Metabol 50(5): 876-883.

Azziz, R., E. Carmina, et al. (2006). "Positions statement: criteria for defining polycystic ovary syndrome as a predominantly hyperandrogenic syndrome: an Androgen Excess Society guideline." J Clin Endocrinol Metab 91(11): 4237-4245.

Azziz, R., D. Ehrmann, et al. (2001). "Troglitazone improves ovulation and hirsutism in the polycystic ovary syndrome: a multicenter, double blind, placebo-controlled trial." J Clin Endocrinol Metab 86(4): 1626-1632.

Baccarelli, A., A. Zanobetti, et al. (2007). "Air pollution, smoking, and plasma homocysteine." Environ Health Perspect 115(2): 176-181.

Baillargeon, J. P., D. J. Jakubowicz, et al. (2004). "Effects of metformin and rosiglitazone, alone and in combination, in nonobese women with polycystic ovary syndrome and normal indices of insulin sensitivity." Fertil Steril 82(4): 893-902.

Balen, A. H., G. S. Conway, et al. (1995). "Polycystic ovary syndrome: the spectrum of the disorder in 1741 patients." Hum Reprod 10(8): 2107-2111.

Banaszewska, B., L. Pawelczyk, et al. (2009). "Comparison of simvastatin and metformin in treatment of polycystic ovary syndrome: prospective randomized trial." J Clin Endocrinol Metab 94(12): 4938-4945.

Baptiste, C. G., M. C. Battista, et al. (2010). "Insulin and hyperandrogenism in women with polycystic ovary syndrome." J Steroid Biochem Mol Biol 122(1-3): 42-52.

Barber, T. M., J. A. Wass, et al. (2007). "Metabolic characteristics of women with polycystic ovaries and oligo-amenorrhoea but normal androgen levels: implications for the management of polycystic ovary syndrome." Clin Endocrinol (Oxf) 66(4): 513-517.

Barbieri, R. L., A. Makris, et al. (1984). "Insulin stimulates androgen accumulation in incubations of human ovarian stroma and theca." Obstet Gynecol 64(3 Suppl): 73S-80S.

Barrett-Connor, E. and D. Goodman-Gruen (1995). "Prospective study of endogenous sex hormones and fatal cardiovascular disease in postmenopausal women." BMJ 311(7014): 1193-1196.

Benson, S., P. C. Arck, et al. (2009). "Disturbed stress responses in women with polycystic ovary syndrome." Psychoneuroendocrinology 34(5): 727-735.

Bernini, G. P., M. Sgro, et al. (1999). "Endogenous androgens and carotid intimal-medial thickness in women." J Clin Endocrinol Metab 84(6): 2008-2012.

Birdsall, M. A., C. M. Farquhar, et al. (1997). "Association between polycystic ovaries and extent of coronary artery disease in women having cardiac catheterization." Ann Intern Med 126(1): 32-35.

Bishop, S. C., S. Basch, et al. (2009). "Polycystic ovary syndrome, depression, and affective disorders." Endocr Pract 15(5): 475-482.

Blankenberg, S., L. Tiret, et al. (2002). "Interleukin-18 is a strong predictor of cardiovascular death in stable and unstable angina." Circulation 106(1): 24-30.

Book, C. B. and A. Dunaif (1999). "Selective insulin resistance in the polycystic ovary syndrome." J Clin Endocrinol Metab 84(9): 3110-3116.

Bots, M. L., J. M. Dijk, et al. (2002). "Carotid intima-media thickness, arterial stiffness and risk of cardiovascular disease: current evidence." J Hypertens 20(12): 2317-2325.

Boulman, N., Y. Levy, et al. (2004). "Increased C-reactive protein levels in the polycystic ovary syndrome: a marker of cardiovascular disease." J Clin Endocrinol Metab 89(5): 2160-2165.

Bremer, A. A. and W. L. Miller (2008). "The serine phosphorylation hypothesis of polycystic ovary syndrome: a unifying mechanism for hyperandrogenemia and insulin resistance." Fertil Steril 89(5): 1039-1048.

Brooks, D., R. L. Horner, et al. (1997). "Obstructive sleep apnea as a cause of systemic hypertension. Evidence from a canine model." J Clin Invest 99(1): 106-109.

Bruner, B., K. Chad, et al. (2006). "Effects of exercise and nutritional counseling in women with polycystic ovary syndrome." Appl Physiol Nutr Metab 31(4): 384-391.

Brunzell, J. D. and A. F. Ayyobi (2003). "Dyslipidemia in the metabolic syndrome and type 2 diabetes mellitus." Am J Med 115 Suppl 8A: 24S-28S.

Brutsaert, D. L., S. U. Sys, et al. (1993). "Diastolic failure: pathophysiology and therapeutic implications." J Am Coll Cardiol 22(1): 318-325.

Burghen, G. A., J. R. Givens, et al. (1980). "Correlation of hyperandrogenism with hyperinsulinism in polycystic ovarian disease." J Clin Endocrinol Metab 50(1): 113-116.

Carmina, E. (2002). "Anti-androgens for the treatment of hirsutism." Expert Opin Investig Drugs 11(3): 357-363

Christian, R. C., D. A. Dumesic, et al. (2003). "Prevalence and predictors of coronary artery calcification in women with polycystic ovary syndrome." J Clin Endocrinol Metab 88(6): 2562-2568.

Ciaraldi, T. P., A. J. Morales, et al. (1998). "Lack of insulin resistance in fibroblasts from subjects with polycystic ovary syndrome." Metabolism 47(8): 940-946.

Cibula, D., R. Cifkova, et al. (2000). "Increased risk of non-insulin dependent diabetes mellitus, arterial hypertension and coronary artery disease in perimenopausal women with a history of the polycystic ovary syndrome." Hum Reprod 15(4): 785-789.

Clark, A. M., W. Ledger, et al. (1995). "Weight loss results in significant improvement in pregnancy and ovulation rates in anovulatory obese women." Hum Reprod 10(10): 2705-2712.

Clayton, R. N., V. Ogden, et al. (1992). "How common are polycystic ovaries in normal women and what is their significance for the fertility of the population?" Clin Endocrinol (Oxf) 37(2): 127-134.

Coetzee, E. J. and W. P. Jackson (1979). "Metformin in management of pregnant insulin-independent diabetics." Diabetologia 16(4): 241-245.

D'Angelo, A., A. Coppola, et al. (2000). "The role of vitamin B12 in fasting hyperhomocysteinemia and its interaction with the homozygous C677T mutation of the methylenetetrahydrofolate reductase (MTHFR) gene. A case-control study of patients with early-onset thrombotic events." Thromb Haemost 83(4): 563-570.

D'Angelo, A. and J. Selhub (1997). "Homocysteine and thrombotic disease." Blood 90(1): 1-11.

Dahlgren, E., P. O. Janson, et al. (1992). "Polycystic ovary syndrome and risk for myocardial infarction. Evaluated from a risk factor model based on a prospective population study of women." Acta Obstet Gynecol Scand 71(8): 599-604.

Dahlgren, E., P. O. Janson, et al. (1994). "Hemostatic and metabolic variables in women with polycystic ovary syndrome." Fertil Steril 61(3): 455-460.

Dahlgren, E., K. Landin, et al. (1998). "Effects of two antiandrogen treatments on hirsutism and insulin sensitivity in women with polycystic ovary syndrome." Hum Reprod 13(1O): 2706-2711.

Dalton, M., A. J. Cameron, et al. (2003). "Waist circumference, waist-hip ratio and body mass index and their correlation with cardiovascular disease risk factors in Australian adults." J Intern Med 254(6): 555-563.

Davi, G., M. T. Guagnano, et al. (2002). "Platelet activation in obese women: role of inflammation and oxidant stress." JAMA 288(16): 2008-2014.

De Backer, G., E. Ambrosioni, et al. (2003). "European guidelines on cardiovascular disease prevention in clinical practice. Third Joint Task Force of European and Other Societies on Cardiovascular Disease Prevention in Clinical Practice." Eur Heart J 24(17): 1601-1610.

Dejager, S., C. Pichard, et al. (2001). "Smaller LDL particle size in women with polycystic ovary syndrome compared to controls." Clin Endocrinol (Oxf) 54(4): 455-462.

de la Calle, M., T. Gallardo, et al. (2007). "[Increased homocysteine levels in polycystic ovary syndrome]." Med Clin (Barc) 129(8): 292-294.

Demirel, F., A. Bideci, et al. (2007). "Serum leptin, oxidized low density lipoprotein and plasma asymmetric dimethylarginine levels and their relationship with dyslipidaemia in adolescent girls with polycystic ovary syndrome." Clin Endocrinol (Oxf) 67(1): 129-134.

Despres, J. P., S. Moorjani, et al. (1990). "Regional distribution of body fat, plasma lipoproteins, and cardiovascular disease." Arteriosclerosis 10(4): 497-511.

Diamanti-Kandarakis, E., K. Alexandraki, et al. (2005). "Metformin administration improves endothelial function in women with polycystic ovary syndrome." Eur J Endocrinol 152(5): 749-756.

Diamanti-Kandarakis, E., C. Kouli, et al. (1998). "Therapeutic effects of metformin on insulin resistance and hyperandrogenism in polycystic ovary syndrome." Eur J Endocrinol 138(3): 269-274.

Diamanti-Kandarakis, E., C. R. Kouli, et al. (1999). "A survey of the polycystic ovary syndrome in the Greek island of Lesbos: hormonal and metabolic profile." J Clin Endocrinol Metab 84(11): 4006-4011.

Diamanti-Kandarakis, E. and A. G. Papavassiliou (2006). "Molecular mechanisms of insulin resistance in polycystic ovary syndrome." Trends Mol Med 12(7): 324-332.

Diamanti-Kandarakis, E., G. Spina, et al. (2001). "Increased endothelin-1 levels in women with polycystic ovary syndrome and the beneficial effect of metformin therapy." J Clin Endocrinol Metab 86(10): 4666-4673.

Dierkes, J., S. Westphal, et al. (2004). "The effect of fibrates and other lipid-lowering drugs on plasma homocysteine levels." Expert Opin Drug Saf 3(2): 101-111.

Duleba, A. J., B. Banaszewska, et al. (2006). "Simvastatin improves biochemical parameters in women with polycystic ovary syndrome: results of a prospective, randomized trial." Fertil Steril 85(4): 996-1001.

Dunaif, A. (1997). "Insulin resistance and the polycystic ovary syndrome: mechanism and implications for pathogenesis." Endocr Rev 18(6): 774-800.

Dunaif, A., D. Scott, et al. (1996). "The insulin-sensitizing agent troglitazone improves metabolic and reproductive abnormalities in the polycystic ovary syndrome." J Clin Endocrinol Metab 81(9): 3299-3306.

Dunaif, A., K. R. Segal, et al. (1989). "Profound peripheral insulin resistance, independent of obesity, in polycystic ovary syndrome." Diabetes 38(9): 1165-1174.

Dyken, M. E., V. K. Somers, et al. (1996). "Investigating the relationship between stroke and obstructive sleep apnea." Stroke 27(3): 401-407.

Ehrmann, D. A. (2005). "Polycystic ovary syndrome." N Engl J Med 352(12): 1223-1236.

Ehrmann, D. A., R. B. Barnes, et al. (1999). "Prevalence of impaired glucose tolerance and diabetes in women with polycystic ovary syndrome." Diabetes Care 22(1): 141-146.

Ehrmann, D. A., J. Sturis, et al. (1995). "Insulin secretory defects in polycystic ovary syndrome. Relationship to insulin sensitivity and family history of non-insulin-dependent diabetes mellitus." J Clin Invest 96(1): 520-527.

Eisner, J. R., M. A. Barnett, et al. (2002). "Ovarian hyperandrogenism in adult female rhesus monkeys exposed to prenatal androgen excess." Fertil Steril 77(1): 167-172.

Elkind-Hirsch, K., O. Marrioneaux, et al. (2008). "Comparison of single and combined treatment with exenatide and metformin on menstrual cyclicity in overweight women with polycystic ovary syndrome." J Clin Endocrinol Metab 93(7): 2670-2678.

Elter, K., G. Imir, et al. (2002). "Clinical, endocrine and metabolic effects of metformin added to ethinyl estradiol-cyproterone acetate in non-obese women with polycystic ovarian syndrome: a randomized controlled study." Hum Reprod 17(7): 1729-1737.

Escobar-Morreale, H. F., G. Villuendas, et al. (2003). "Obesity, and not insulin resistance, is the major determinant of serum inflammatory cardiovascular risk markers in pre-menopausal women." Diabetologia 46(5): 625-633.

Essah, P. A., J. E. Nestler, et al. (2008). "Differences in dyslipidemia between American and Italian women with polycystic ovary syndrome." J Endocrinol Invest 31(1): 35-41.

Fermo, I., S. Vigano' D'Angelo, et al. (1995). "Prevalence of moderate hyperhomocysteinemia in patients with early-onset venous and arterial occlusive disease." Ann Intern Med 123(10): 747-753.

Ferrannini, E., A. Natali, et al. (1997). "Insulin resistance and hypersecretion in obesity. European Group for the Study of Insulin Resistance (EGIR)." J Clin Invest 100(5): 1166-1173.

Fogel, R. B., A. Malhotra, et al. (2001). "Increased prevalence of obstructive sleep apnea syndrome in obese women with polycystic ovary syndrome." J Clin Endocrinol Metab 86(3): 1175-1180.

Franks, S. (1995). "Polycystic ovary syndrome." N Engl J Med 333(13): 853-861.

Franks, S., D. Kiddy, et al. (1991). "Obesity and polycystic ovary syndrome." Ann N Y Acad Sci 626: 201-206.

Gardner, C. D., S. P. Fortmann, et al. (1996). "Association of small low-density lipoprotein particles with the incidence of coronary artery disease in men and women." JAMA 276(11): 875-881.

Glintborg, D., K. Hojlund, et al. (2008). "Soluble CD36 and risk markers of insulin resistance and atherosclerosis are elevated in polycystic ovary syndrome and significantly reduced during pioglitazone treatment." Diabetes Care 31(2): 328-334.

Gorgels, W. J., Y. v d Graaf, et al. (1997). "Urinary sex hormone excretions in premenopausal women and coronary heart disease risk: a nested case-referent study in the DOM-cohort." J Clin Epidemiol 50(3): 275-281.

Guzick, D. S. (2004). "Cardiovascular risk in PCOS." J Clin Endocrinol Metab 89(8): 3694-3695.

Guzick, D. S., E. O. Talbott, et al. (1996). "Carotid atherosclerosis in women with polycystic ovary syndrome: initial results from a case-control study." Am J Obstet Gynecol 174(4): 1224-1229; discussion 1229-1232.

Guzick, D. S., R. Wing, et al. (1994). "Endocrine consequences of weight loss in obese, hyperandrogenic, anovulatory women." Fertil Steril 61(4): 598-604.

Hatch, R., R. L. Rosenfield, et al. (1981). "Hirsutism: implications, etiology, and management." Am J Obstet Gynecol 140(7): 815-830.

Hines, G., C. Moran, et al. (2001). "Facial and abdominal hair growth in hirsutism: a computerized evaluation." J Am Acad Dermatol 45(6): 846-850.

Hollinrake, E., A. Abreu, et al. (2007). "Increased risk of depressive disorders in women with polycystic ovary syndrome." Fertil Steril 87(6): 1369-1376.

Holte, J., T. Bergh, et al. (1995). "Restored insulin sensitivity but persistently increased early insulin secretion after weight loss in obese women with polycystic ovary syndrome." J Clin Endocrinol Metab 80(9): 2586-2593.

Homburg, R. (1996). "Polycystic ovary syndrome - from gynaecological curiosity to multisystem endocrinopathy." Hum Reprod 11(1): 29-39.

Hotamisligil, G. S., N. S. Shargill, et al. (1993). "Adipose expression of tumor necrosis factor-alpha: direct role in obesity-linked insulin resistance." Science 259(5091): 87-91.

Hung, J., E. G. Whitford, et al. (1990). "Association of sleep apnoea with myocardial infarction in men." Lancet 336(8710): 261-264.

Jedel, E., M. Waern, et al. (2010). "Anxiety and depression symptoms in women with polycystic ovary syndrome compared with controls matched for body mass index." Hum Reprod 25(2): 450-456.

Jones, G. L., J. M. Hall, et al. (2008). "Health-related quality of life measurement in women with polycystic ovary syndrome: a systematic review." Hum Reprod Update 14(1): 15-25.

Kelly, C. C., H. Lyall, et al. (2001). "Low grade chronic inflammation in women with polycystic ovarian syndrome." J Clin Endocrinol Metab 86(6): 2453-2455.

Kelly, C. J., A. Speirs, et al. (2002). "Altered vascular function in young women with polycystic ovary syndrome." J Clin Endocrinol Metab 87(2): 742-746.

Kiddy, D. S., D. Hamilton-Fairley, et al. (1992). "Improvement in endocrine and ovarian function during dietary treatment of obese women with polycystic ovary syndrome." Clin Endocrinol (Oxf) 36(1): 105-111.

Kiddy, D. S., D. Hamilton-Fairley, et al. (1989). "Diet-induced changes in sex hormone binding globulin and free testosterone in women with normal or polycystic ovaries: correlation with serum insulin and insulin-like growth factor-I." Clin Endocrinol (Oxf) 31(6): 757-763.

Kiddy, D. S., P. S. Sharp, et al. (1990). "Differences in clinical and endocrine features between obese and non-obese subjects with polycystic ovary syndrome: an analysis of 263 consecutive cases." Clin Endocrinol (Oxf) 32(2): 213-220.

Knochenhauer, E. S., T. J. Key, et al. (1998). "Prevalence of the polycystic ovary syndrome in unselected black and white women of the southeastern United States: a prospective study." J Clin Endocrinol Metab 83(9): 3078-3082.

Kodaman, P. H. and A. J. Duleba (2008). "Statins in the treatment of polycystic ovary syndrome." Semin Reprod Med 26(1): 127-138.

Korhonen, S., M. Hippelainen, et al. (2001). "Relationship of the metabolic syndrome and obesity to polycystic ovary syndrome: a controlled, population-based study." Am J Obstet Gynecol 184(3): 289-296.

Korytkowski, M. T., M. Mokan, et al. (1995). "Metabolic effects of oral contraceptives in women with polycystic ovary syndrome." J Clin Endocrinol Metab 80(11): 3327-3334.

Kuczmarski, R. J., K. M. Flegal, et al. (1994). "Increasing prevalence of overweight among US adults. The National Health and Nutrition Examination Surveys, 1960 to 1991." JAMA 272(3): 205-211.

Kumada, M., S. Kihara, et al. (2003). "Association of hypoadiponectinemia with coronary artery disease in men." Arterioscler Thromb Vasc Biol 23(1): 85-89.

Lakhani, K., N. Constantinovici, et al. (2000). "Internal carotid artery haemodynamics in women with polycystic ovaries." Clin Sci (Lond) 98(6): 661-665.

Lavie, P., P. Herer, et al. (2000). "Obstructive sleep apnoea syndrome as a risk factor for hypertension: population study." BMJ 320(7233): 479-482.

Legro, R. S., C. L. Gnatuk, et al. (2005). "Changes in glucose tolerance over time in women with polycystic ovary syndrome: a controlled study." J Clin Endocrinol Metab 90(6): 3236-3242.

Legro, R. S., A. R. Kunselman, et al. (1999). "Prevalence and predictors of risk for type 2 diabetes mellitus and impaired glucose tolerance in polycystic ovary syndrome: a prospective, controlled study in 254 affected women." J Clin Endocrinol Metab 84(1): 165-169.

Legro, R. S., A. R. Kunselman, et al. (2001). "Prevalence and predictors of dyslipidemia in women with polycystic ovary syndrome." Am J Med 111(8): 607-613.

Lindsay, R. S., T. Funahashi, et al. (2002). "Adiponectin and development of type 2 diabetes in the Pima Indian population." Lancet 360(9326): 57-58.

Lo, J. C., S. L. Feigenbaum, et al. (2006). "Epidemiology and adverse cardiovascular risk profile of diagnosed polycystic ovary syndrome." J Clin Endocrinol Metab 91(4): 1357-1363.

London, G. M., S. J. Marchais, et al. (2004). "Arterial stiffness and function in end-stage renal disease." Adv Chronic Kidney Dis 11(2): 202-209.

Lookingbill, D. P., L. M. Demers, et al. (1991). "Clinical and biochemical parameters of androgen action in normal healthy Caucasian versus Chinese subjects." J Clin Endocrinol Metab 72(6): 1242-1248.

Loverro, G., F. Lorusso, et al. (2002). "The plasma homocysteine levels are increased in polycystic ovary syndrome." Gynecol Obstet Invest 53(3): 157-162.

Luque-Ramirez, M., F. Alvarez-Blasco, et al. (2007). "Obesity is the major determinant of the abnormalities in blood pressure found in young women with the polycystic ovary syndrome." J Clin Endocrinol Metab 92(6): 2141-2148.

Maitra, A., R. R. Pingle, et al. (2001). "Dyslipidemia with particular regard to apolipoprotein profile in association with polycystic ovary syndrome: a study among Indian women." Int J Fertil Womens Med 46(5): 271-277.

Manneras-Holm, L., F. Baghaei, et al. (2011). "Coagulation and fibrinolytic disturbances in women with polycystic ovary syndrome." J Clin Endocrinol Metab 96(4): 1068-1076.

Manson, J. E., G. A. Colditz, et al. (1990). "A prospective study of obesity and risk of coronary heart disease in women." N Engl J Med 322(13): 882-889.

Masi, A. T., S. L. Feigenbaum, et al. (1995). "Hormonal and pregnancy relationships to rheumatoid arthritis: convergent effects with immunologic and microvascular systems." Semin Arthritis Rheum 25(1): 1-27.

Mather, K. J., F. Kwan, et al. (2000). "Hyperinsulinemia in polycystic ovary syndrome correlates with increased cardiovascular risk independent of obesity." Fertil Steril 73(1): 150-156.

Mayer, E. L., D. W. Jacobsen, et al. (1996). "Homocysteine and coronary atherosclerosis." J Am Coll Cardiol 27(3): 517-527.

Meyer, C., B. P. McGrath, et al. (2005). "Vascular dysfunction and metabolic parameters in polycystic ovary syndrome." J Clin Endocrinol Metab 90(8): 4630-4635.

Moghetti, P., R. Castello, et al. (2000). "Metformin effects on clinical features, endocrine and metabolic profiles, and insulin sensitivity in polycystic ovary syndrome: a randomized, double-blind, placebo-controlled 6-month trial, followed by open, long-term clinical evaluation." J Clin Endocrinol Metab 85(1): 139-146.

Mohlig, M., J. Spranger, et al. (2004). "The polycystic ovary syndrome per se is not associated with increased chronic inflammation." Eur J Endocrinol 150(4): 525-532.

Moran, L. J., R. Pasquali, et al. (2009). "Treatment of obesity in polycystic ovary syndrome: a position statement of the Androgen Excess and Polycystic Ovary Syndrome Society." Fertil Steril 92(6): 1966-1982.

Morin-Papunen, L., K. Rautio, et al. (2003). "Metformin reduces serum C-reactive protein levels in women with polycystic ovary syndrome." J Clin Endocrinol Metab 88(10): 4649-4654.

Morin-Papunen, L. C., I. Vauhkonen, et al. (2000). "Endocrine and metabolic effects of metformin versus ethinyl estradiol-cyproterone acetate in obese women with polycystic ovary syndrome: a randomized study." J Clin Endocrinol Metab 85(9): 3161-3168.

Nagayama, M., Y. Shinohara, et al. (1994). "Lipoprotein(a) and ischemic cerebrovascular disease in young adults." Stroke 25(1): 74-78.

Nelson-Degrave, V. L., J. K. Wickenheisser, et al. (2005). "Alterations in mitogen-activated protein kinase kinase and extracellular regulated kinase signaling in theca cells contribute to excessive androgen production in polycystic ovary syndrome." Mol Endocrinol 19(2): 379-390.

Nieuwenhuis-Ruifrok, A. E., W. K. Kuchenbecker, et al. (2009). "Insulin sensitizing drugs for weight loss in women of reproductive age who are overweight or obese: systematic review and meta-analysis." Hum Reprod Update 15(1): 57-68.

Nishizawa, H., I. Shimomura, et al. (2002). "Androgens decrease plasma adiponectin, an insulin-sensitizing adipocyte-derived protein." Diabetes 51(9): 2734-2741.

Nitsche, K. and D. A. Ehrmann (2010). "Obstructive sleep apnea and metabolic dysfunction in polycystic ovary syndrome." Best Pract Res Clin Endocrinol Metab 24(5): 717-730.

Norman, R. J., M. J. Davies, et al. (2002). "The role of lifestyle modification in polycystic ovary syndrome." Trends Endocrinol Metab 13(6): 251-257.

Norman, R. J., L. Masters, et al. (2001). "Relative risk of conversion from normoglycaemia to impaired glucose tolerance or non-insulin dependent diabetes mellitus in polycystic ovarian syndrome." Hum Reprod 16(9): 1995-1998.

Norman, R. J., S. C. Masters, et al. (1995). "Metabolic approaches to the subclassification of polycystic ovary syndrome." Fertil Steril 63(2): 329-335.

Okajima, T., T. Koyanagi, et al. (1994). "[Hormonal abnormalities were improved by weight loss using very low calorie diet in a patient with polycystic ovary syndrome]." Fukuoka Igaku Zasshi 85(9): 263-266.

Oktem, M., E. E. Ozcimen, et al. (2009). "Polycystic ovary syndrome is associated with elevated plasma soluble CD40 ligand, a marker of coronary artery disease." Fertil Steril 91(6): 2545-2550.

Orio, F., Jr., S. Palomba, et al. (2005). "The increase of leukocytes as a new putative marker of low-grade chronic inflammation and early cardiovascular risk in polycystic ovary syndrome." J Clin Endocrinol Metab 90(1): 2-5.

Orio, F., Jr., S. Palomba, et al. (2004). "Early impairment of endothelial structure and function in young normal-weight women with polycystic ovary syndrome." J Clin Endocrinol Metab 89(9): 4588-4593.

Orio, F., Jr., S. Palomba, et al. (2004). "The cardiovascular risk of young women with polycystic ovary syndrome: an observational, analytical, prospective case-control study." J Clin Endocrinol Metab 89(8): 3696-3701.

Orio, F., Jr., S. Palomba, et al. (2003). "Homocysteine levels and C677T polymorphism of methylenetetrahydrofolate reductase in women with polycystic ovary syndrome." J Clin Endocrinol Metab 88(2): 673-679.

Ouchi, N., S. Kihara, et al. (2003). "Reciprocal association of C-reactive protein with adiponectin in blood stream and adipose tissue." Circulation 107(5): 671-674.

Ounpuu, S., A. Negassa, et al. (2001). "INTER-HEART: A global study of risk factors for acute myocardial infarction." Am Heart J 141(5): 711-721.

Panidis, D., A. Kourtis, et al. (2003). "Serum adiponectin levels in women with polycystic ovary syndrome." Hum Reprod 18(9): 1790-1796.

Paradisi, G., H. O. Steinberg, et al. (2003). "Troglitazone therapy improves endothelial function to near normal levels in women with polycystic ovary syndrome." J Clin Endocrinol Metab 88(2): 576-580.

Paradisi, G., H. O. Steinberg, et al. (2001). "Polycystic ovary syndrome is associated with endothelial dysfunction." Circulation 103(10): 1410-1415.

Pessin, J. E. and A. R. Saltiel (2000). "Signaling pathways in insulin action: molecular targets of insulin resistance." J Clin Invest 106(2): 165-169.

Pirwany, I. R., R. Fleming, et al. (2001). "Lipids and lipoprotein subfractions in women with PCOS: relationship to metabolic and endocrine parameters." Clin Endocrinol (Oxf) 54(4): 447-453.

Poretsky, L., N. A. Cataldo, et al. (1999). "The insulin-related ovarian regulatory system in health and disease." Endocr Rev 20(4): 535-582.

Price, J. F., A. J. Lee, et al. (1997). "Steroid sex hormones and peripheral arterial disease in the Edinburgh Artery Study." Steroids 62(12): 789-794.

Puder, J. J., S. Varga, et al. (2005). "Central fat excess in polycystic ovary syndrome: relation to low-grade inflammation and insulin resistance." J Clin Endocrinol Metab 90(11): 6014-6021.

Rautio, K., J. S. Tapanainen, et al. (2005). "Effects of metformin and ethinyl estradiol-cyproterone acetate on lipid levels in obese and non-obese women with polycystic ovary syndrome." Eur J Endocrinol 152(2): 269-275.
Rebora, A. (2001). "Baldness and coronary artery disease: the dermatologic point of view of a controversial issue." Arch Dermatol 137(7): 943-947.
Rizzo, M., K. Berneis, et al. (2008). "How should we manage atherogenic dyslipidemia in women with polycystic ovary syndrome?" Am J Obstet Gynecol 198(1): 28 e21-25
Rizzo, M., K. Berneis, et al. (2009). "Milder forms of atherogenic dyslipidemia in ovulatory versus anovulatory polycystic ovary syndrome phenotype." Hum Reprod 24(9): 2286-2292.
Rose, G. (1981). "Strategy of prevention: lessons from cardiovascular disease." Br Med J (Clin Res Ed) 282(6279): 1847-1851.
Rosenbaum, M., R. L. Leibel, et al. (1997). "Obesity." N Engl J Med 337(6): 396-407.
Rosenzweig, J. L., E. Ferrannini, et al. (2008). "Primary prevention of cardiovascular disease and type 2 diabetes in patients at metabolic risk: an endocrine society clinical practice guideline." J Clin Endocrinol Metab 93(10): 3671-3689.
Sabuncu, T., H. Vural, et al. (2001). "Oxidative stress in polycystic ovary syndrome and its contribution to the risk of cardiovascular disease." Clin Biochem 34(5): 407-413.
Sandkamp, M., H. Funke, et al. (1990). "Lipoprotein(a) is an independent risk factor for myocardial infarction at a young age." Clin Chem 36(1): 20-23.
Sathyapalan, T., E. S. Kilpatrick, et al. (2009). "The effect of atorvastatin in patients with polycystic ovary syndrome: a randomized double-blind placebo-controlled study." J Clin Endocrinol Metab 94(1): 103-108.
Schannwell, C. M., M. Schneppenheim, et al. (2002). "Left ventricular diastolic dysfunction as an early manifestation of diabetic cardiomyopathy." Cardiology 98(1-2): 33-39.
Scanu, A. M. (1992). "Lipoprotein(a). A genetic risk factor for premature coronary heart disease." JAMA 267(24): 3326-3329.
Scarpitta, A. M. and D. Sinagra (2000). "Polycystic ovary syndrome: an endocrine and metabolic disease." Gynecol Endocrinol 14(5): 392-395.
Shahar, E., S. Redline, et al. (2003). "Hormone replacement therapy and sleep-disordered breathing." Am J Respir Crit Care Med 167(9): 1186-1192.
Sharma, S. T., E. P. Wickham, 3rd, et al. (2007). "Changes in glucose tolerance with metformin treatment in polycystic ovary syndrome: a retrospective analysis." Endocr Pract 13(4): 373-379.
Schillaci, G., L. Pasqualini, et al. (2002). "Prognostic significance of left ventricular diastolic dysfunction in essential hypertension." J Am Coll Cardiol 39(12): 2005-2011.
Shaw, L. J., C. N. Bairey Merz, et al. (2008). "Postmenopausal women with a history of irregular menses and elevated androgen measurements at high risk for worsening cardiovascular event-free survival: results from the National Institutes of Health--National Heart, Lung, and Blood Institute sponsored Women's Ischemia Syndrome Evaluation." J Clin Endocrinol Metab 93(4): 1276-1284.
Shroff, R., A. Kerchner, et al. (2007). "Young obese women with polycystic ovary syndrome have evidence of early coronary atherosclerosis." J Clin Endocrinol Metab 92(12): 4609-4614.
Spranger, J., M. Mohlig, et al. (2004). "Adiponectin is independently associated with insulin sensitivity in women with polycystic ovary syndrome." Clin Endocrinol (Oxf) 61(6): 738-746.

Stein, I. F. and M. L. Leventhal. (1935). " Amenorrhoea associated with bilateral polycystic ovaries. " Am. J. Obstet. Gynecol: 181-191.
Stephens, J. M., M. D. Butts, et al. (1992). "Regulation of transcription factor mRNA accumulation during 3T3-L1 preadipocyte differentiation by tumour necrosis factor-alpha." J Mol Endocrinol 9(1): 61-72.
Stramba-Badiale, M., K. M. Fox, et al. (2006). "Cardiovascular diseases in women: a statement from the policy conference of the European Society of Cardiology." Eur Heart J 27(8): 994-1005.
Sverrisdottir, Y. B., T. Mogren, et al. (2008). "Is polycystic ovary syndrome associated with high sympathetic nerve activity and size at birth?" Am J Physiol Endocrinol Metab 294(3): E576-581.
Talbott, E., A. Clerici, et al. (1998). "Adverse lipid and coronary heart disease risk profiles in young women with polycystic ovary syndrome: results of a case-control study." J Clin Epidemiol 51(5): 415-422.
Talbott, E. O., D. S. Guzick, et al. (2000). "Evidence for association between polycystic ovary syndrome and premature carotid atherosclerosis in middle-aged women." Arterioscler Thromb Vasc Biol 20(11): 2414-2421.
Talbott, E., D. Guzick, et al. (1995). "Coronary heart disease risk factors in women with polycystic ovary syndrome." Arterioscler Thromb Vasc Biol 15(7): 821-826.
Talbott, E. O., J. V. Zborowski, et al. (2004). "Evidence for an association between metabolic cardiovascular syndrome and coronary and aortic calcification among women with polycystic ovary syndrome." J Clin Endocrinol Metab 89(11): 5454-5461.
Tan, K. C., A. Xu, et al. (2004). "Hypoadiponectinemia is associated with impaired endothelium-dependent vasodilation." J Clin Endocrinol Metab 89(2): 765-769.
Taponen, S., H. Martikainen, et al. (2004). "Metabolic cardiovascular disease risk factors in women with self-reported symptoms of oligomenorrhea and/or hirsutism: Northern Finland Birth Cohort 1966 Study." J Clin Endocrinol Metab 89(5): 2114-2118.
Tarkun, I., B. Cetinarslan, et al. (2005). "Effect of rosiglitazone on insulin resistance, C-reactive protein and endothelial function in non-obese young women with polycystic ovary syndrome." Eur J Endocrinol 153(1): 115-121.
Thomson, R. L., J. D. Buckley, et al. (2010). "Lifestyle management improves quality of life and depression in overweight and obese women with polycystic ovary syndrome." Fertil Steril 94(5): 1812-1816.
Tiras, M. B., R. Yalcin, et al. (1999). "Alterations in cardiac flow parameters in patients with polycystic ovarian syndrome." Hum Reprod 14(8): 1949-1952.
Toulis, K. A., D. G. Goulis, et al. (2011). "Meta-analysis of cardiovascular disease risk markers in women with polycystic ovary syndrome." Hum Reprod Update.
Trolle, B., A. Flyvbjerg, et al. (2007). "Efficacy of metformin in obese and non-obese women with polycystic ovary syndrome: a randomized, double-blinded, placebo-controlled cross-over trial." Hum Reprod 22(11): 2967-2973.
Tsilchorozidou, T., C. Overton, et al. (2004). "The pathophysiology of polycystic ovary syndrome." Clin Endocrinol (Oxf) 60(1): 1-17.
Valkenburg, O., R. P. Steegers-Theunissen, et al. (2008). "A more atherogenic serum lipoprotein profile is present in women with polycystic ovary syndrome: a case-control study." J Clin Endocrinol Metab 93(2): 470-476.

van Kesteren, P. J., H. Asscheman, et al. (1997). "Mortality and morbidity in transsexual subjects treated with cross-sex hormones." Clin Endocrinol (Oxf) 47(3): 337-342.

Velazquez, E., A. Acosta, et al. (1997). "Menstrual cyclicity after metformin therapy in polycystic ovary syndrome." Obstet Gynecol 90(3): 392-395.

Vgontzas, A. N., R. S. Legro, et al. (2001). "Polycystic ovary syndrome is associated with obstructive sleep apnea and daytime sleepiness: role of insulin resistance." J Clin Endocrinol Metab 86(2): 517-520.

Vigorito, C., F. Giallauria, et al. (2007). "Beneficial effects of a three-month structured exercise training program on cardiopulmonary functional capacity in young women with polycystic ovary syndrome." J Clin Endocrinol Metab 92(4): 1379-1384.

Wild, R. A., P. C. Painter, et al. (1985). "Lipoprotein lipid concentrations and cardiovascular risk in women with polycystic ovary syndrome." J Clin Endocrinol Metab 61(5): 946-951.

Wild, S., T. Pierpoint, et al. (2000). "Cardiovascular disease in women with polycystic ovary syndrome at long-term follow-up: a retrospective cohort study." Clin Endocrinol (Oxf) 52(5): 595-600.

Vryonidou, A., A. Papatheodorou, et al. (2005). "Association of hyperandrogenemic and metabolic phenotype with carotid intima-media thickness in young women with polycystic ovary syndrome." J Clin Endocrinol Metab 90(5): 2740-2746.

Vural, B., E. Caliskan, et al. (2005). "Evaluation of metabolic syndrome frequency and premature carotid atherosclerosis in young women with polycystic ovary syndrome." Hum Reprod 20(9): 2409-2413.

Wierzbicki, A. S. (2008). "Lipoproteins: from A to B and maybe C-III." Int J Clin Pract 62(5): 674-676.

Wild, R. A., B. Grubb, et al. (1990). "Clinical signs of androgen excess as risk factors for coronary artery disease." Fertil Steril 54(2): 255-259.

Wu, F. C. and A. von Eckardstein (2003). "Androgens and coronary artery disease." Endocr Rev 24(2): 183-217.

Yilmaz, N., M. Pektas, et al. (2008). "The correlation of plasma homocysteine with insulin resistance in polycystic ovary syndrome." J Obstet Gynaecol Res 34(3): 384-391.

Zambon, A. and K. Cusi (2007). "The role of fenofibrate in clinical practice." Diab Vasc Dis Res 4 Suppl 3: S15-20.

Zawadzki, J. K. and A. Dunaif (1992). " Diagnostic criteria for polycystic ovary syndrome: towards a rational approach. In: Dunaif A, Givens JR, Haseltine FP, Merriam GR, editors. Polycystic Ovary Syndrome. Vol. IV. Boston: Blackwell Scientific Publications.": 377-384.

Zhang, L. H., H. Rodriguez, et al. (1995). "Serine phosphorylation of human P450c17 increases 17,20-lyase activity: implications for adrenarche and the polycystic ovary syndrome." Proc Natl Acad Sci U S A 92(23): 10619-10623.

8

Polycystic Ovary Syndrome in the Non-Gynaecological Practice – Can We Use a Common Medical Approach?

Gyula Petrányi
Private medical practice in Internal Medicine, Endocrinology, Diabetes, and Metabolic Diseases, Limassol
Cyprus

1. Introduction

During a recent high-level endocrinology congress, the session on the polycystic ovary syndrome (PCOS) included a lecture on fertility problems. This was started with a remark that the gynaecologist and other medical professionals should bring their treatment efforts closer. I was glad to hear this but thereafter the lecturer talked exclusively about ovulation induction and in vitro fertilisation; and did not say anything about how these efforts affected other medical problems related to PCOS, or the future course of the disease, or what else could be done if the discussed fertility approaches fail (in a high proportion of cases). Why then did he call attention to bringing treatment protocols closer?

Somebody remarked that in their experience even a few months' pre-treatment with metformin improved the results but this was rebuffed by the lecturer that such efforts had not reached sound evidence. After the session, I asked him in private if his patients should have been treated for other existing problems beyond infertility like acne, hirsutism or obesity. The answer was short "They didn't complain about anything else" and he turned his back to me. Well, in all likelihood the patients must have had some hyperandrogenic symptoms as a prerequisite of the diagnosis. In addition, most published fertility studies in the PCOS literature include grossly obese patients. Since obesity alone is a well known contributor to infertility; would be wiser to wait until these women slim down... we have not come closer.

I was a bit angry for not having been taken seriously but it was not the first time I experienced a similar attitude. The patients with irregular periods usually visit the gynaecologist. The general advice that follows is the use of the contraceptive pill if the lady is not interested in becoming pregnant at the moment; or the pharmaceutical stimulation of the ovaries or the laparoscopic drilling to remove the cysts from them if the lady desires a baby.

I bring forth a story of a young girl. Eleni has no plans to get pregnant for years so upon the gynaecologist's advice she starts taking the pill. Her acne spots (all teenagers have pimples, haven't they) and some ugly hairs under her nose were not mentioned and were not commented on either during the visit. Since she doesn't remember or it had not been explained for how long the pills should be taken, she stops the pill after a year or so. She has no boyfriend; the pill might have caused side effects. Despite her spots decreasing and having to remove hair from her face less frequently while on the pill, she gained more weight, interestingly, mainly around the waistline. Was it this why she has not attracted the boys? Off the pill, the annoying spots and hair growth return and the weight gain continues. Slowly she becomes more and more depressed and experiences sudden attacks urging her to take some chocolate or other sweets every now and again. She visits cosmeticians, dermatologists, and dieticians - everything in vain: the problems do not get solved; symptoms come back worsened.

Nobody mentions the suspicion of a chronic disorder that would require a different treatment approach. The irregularity of the periods persists but it is not a disturbing phenomenon; if she visits the gynaecologist, the answer is the same as before. Eventually Eleni gets married and despite making love unprotected for years she is still not pregnant. In desperation she visits fertility clinics where courses of medication are started in increasing doses. Sometimes she gets pregnant but the pregnancy is lost early; on other occasions the medication must be stopped due to dangerous side effects. After six months of ineffective stimulation more complicated and costly in vitro fertilization procedures follow. She is fortunate, with the aid of some further hormonal treatment, the pregnancy goes ahead. She gains more weight than she ought to, there is some fuzz about her elevating blood sugar, she hardly escapes insulin treatment. She can't deliver *per vias naturales* - Caesarean section is required for the oversized but otherwise healthy baby girl. Eleni is now more obese than ever, the menstrual cycles are just as irregular as before pregnancy, and she wonders what problems are inherited by this lovely creature from her.

Dozens of similar stories can be heard from overall the world. Nobody raises the suspicion that thousands of young women might have a very common endocrine-metabolic disorder that can be supposed from the very beginning by a proper look at them and by listening to their medical history?

Without meaning to exaggerate issues, this is a very grim picture. Every article on PCOS starts with the statement that this is the most common endocrine disorder. Despite the prevalence varying according to the diagnostic criteria, it is around 10% of the fertile female population (Azziz et al., 2004; March et al., 2010). PCOS is grossly under-recorded and insufficiently diagnosed in primary care - data from a well-developed country with widely respected health care (Mani et al., 2010).

When one thinks of PCOS, the diagnostic procedure looks complicated and the therapy advice is ambiguous. Usually the treatment options are listed according to the symptoms or explicitly state to start with the main complain of the patient. This is controversial as patients' considerations about their health problems may differ significantly from those regarded important in medical experience.

The most recent review of the American College of Physicians says "Drug therapy is aimed at treating the symptoms of PCOS ... If infertility is not the primary concern, then treatment is aimed at reducing the undesired effects of excess androgen and restoring regular menses to prevent endometrial hyperplasia" (Wilson, 2011). Does this mean that if infertility is the primary concern, nothing else matters? We don't treat tuberculosis only for cough or fever that could be the "primary concern" of the infected. Wherever possible, we use aetiopathogenetic treatment.

Something is missing from the general conception. The advice is definitely misunderstood by those who take it word by word and provide treatment to PCOS patients according to the patient's complain only. Shouldn't we give her the complete information about the nature of the problem with all possible late complications in order that *salus aegroti* will meet *voluntas aegroti* to avoid medico-legal confrontation?

Fortunately, the above cited review on PCOS (Wilson, 2011) says in the third paragraph at the beginning: "The information contained herein should never be used as a substitute for clinical judgment." I agree totally with this statement as it supports my concerns. However, my views will be detailed later in this chapter.

Around 1993 Roy Homburg addressed a lecture on PCOS to the endocrinologists in Cyprus in which he interestingly stated that PCOS had an insulin resistance component in the background; and he advised to start co-cyprindiol (a contraceptive pill containing ethinyloestradiol and ciproterone acetate, a contraceptive combination with anti-androgenic effect which had already been in use on this side of the Atlantic for long) as soon as PCOS is diagnosed to regulate menstruation and to counteract hyperandrogenism; this way preventing progression of the disease. Despite the last part of this opinion being debatable, this lecture raised my curiosity. I started seeing patients with PCOS from this point of view. In the meanwhile the addition of the insulin sensitizer metformin to the treatment repertoire boosted my interest.

Now, nearly two decades on, several substantial aspects of PCOS have still remained unclear (Pasquali et al., 2011). In this chapter only the practical clinical approach to PCOS will be discussed comparing my experience with that of others known from the literature; arguing for a positive answer to the question raised in the chapter title.

2. Diagnostic problems: What is PCOS?

Until the exact pathomechanism is not fully explored PCOS will remain a syndrome: a rather diverse configuration of several endocrine-metabolic features of variable severity.

2.1 Contrasting diagnostic criteria

There have been three recently proposed sets of diagnostic criteria: those of the National Institutes of Health, the NIH criteria (NIH, 1991, as cited in The Rotterdam ESHRE/ASRM-sponsored PCOS consensus workshop group, 2004); the Rotterdam criteria (The Rotterdam ESHRE/ASRM-sponsored PCOS consensus workshop group, 2004); and The Androgen Excess and PCOS Society, the AES criteria (Azziz et al., 2009). They differ in what positive findings are required for the diagnosis but agreed in one: other related (mainly endocrine) disorders must be excluded. I start with a short comment on this statement.

2.1.1 Exclusion of other related disorders

Even this common part of the diagnostic criteria may confuse the unwary. Most endocrine diseases present with symptoms found in PCOS (hyperandrogenic signs, infertility, polycystic ovaries, insulin resistance etc.) but PCOS has no discriminative diagnostic symptoms (none has been found yet) hence the differentiation from other endocrine diseases must be an essential part of the diagnostic procedure. The problem is that PCOS is so frequent (whatever criteria are used) that merely on statistical grounds the same person may suffer from another endocrine disease synchronously.

How can this controversy between the diagnostic criteria and the probability of co-existence of PCOS with another endocrine disorder be solved? It must be obvious that the exclusion statement is meant to say this: any positively diagnosed endocrine disease should be controlled satisfactorily and if the criteria for PCOS still apply one can conclude that the same person suffers also from PCOS.

This coincides with the necessary medical steps emerging from the findings of the diagnostic procedure. Usually the "other" endocrine disorder is of more progressive or dangerous nature than PCOS and its treatment must have priority over PCOS. In consequence, the exclusion criterion would be more equivocal sounding like this: "PCOS exists (if the required diagnostic features apply) with the exclusion of other *uncontrolled* related disorders." Definitions must be robust but equivocal; ambiguity causes hesitation.

Most often hypothyroidism, hyperprolactinaemia or late-onset adrenocortical hyperplasia may coincide with PCOS. Less frequent but more dangerous conditions in the initial phase may also cause problems in the diagnostic procedure.

2.1.2 Positive findings required for the diagnosis

The real debate has been on what positive findings should be included in the diagnostic criteria. There are three main features in question: hyperandrogenism (HA), chronic oligo-anovulation (ANO), and the polycystic appearance of the ovaries on ultrasound (PCO).

The PCO sign was not included in the NIH criteria. The Rotterdam criteria include all three features of which at least two must be present. Later several participants of the Rotterdam consensus meeting realised that hyperandrogenism (androgen excess) is an essential part of PCOS; and their new proposal became known as the AES criteria. This joins ANO and/or PCO in one term, ovarian dysfunction (OD); and PCOS is a combination of HA and OD. In other terms, the combination of PCOS and ANO without HA (one possibility allowed by the Rotterdam criteria) should not be regarded as PCOS. Hyperandrogenism and ovarian dysfunction may not be independent contributors to the development of PCOS but the discussion of this is beyond the scope of this chapter.

2.2 Understanding the differences in the three sets of criteria

The differences of the different diagnostic criteria can be perceived easier using Venn diagrams. Circles represent the population suffering from features specified in the Rotterdam criteria (HA, ANO, and PCO). The overlapping areas (the intersections) of the circles mean the set of people with the common features.

For didactic reasons let us start with the Rotterdam criteria (Fig. 1). The trilobate gray area represents patients who meet at least two of the three possible features; the central pseudo-circle (the intersection of all three circles) includes those who have all three features.

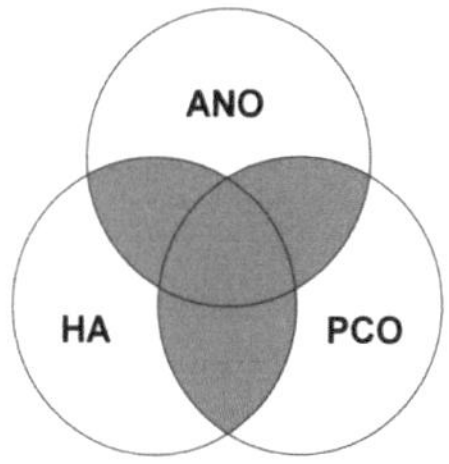

Fig. 1. Visual representation of the patient population diagnosed using the Rotterdam criteria

The gray coloured area in Fig. 2 shows the patients diagnosed by the AES criteria. Ovarian dysfunction is the union of ANO and PCO (and/or). Those who have no hyperandrogenism (the intersection of ANO and PCO less HA) are excluded from the diagnosis.

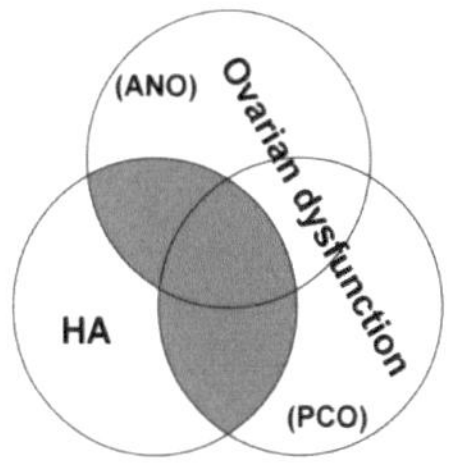

Fig. 2. Visual representation of the patient population diagnosed using the AES criteria

Patients diagnosed by the NIH criteria are those who have both HA and ANO (the intersection of HA and ANO); see in Fig. 3. The PCO sign plays no role in the diagnosis; its inclusion in the diagram is solely for comparative purposes. The number of patients found with PCOS using these NIH criteria is the smallest among the three sets.

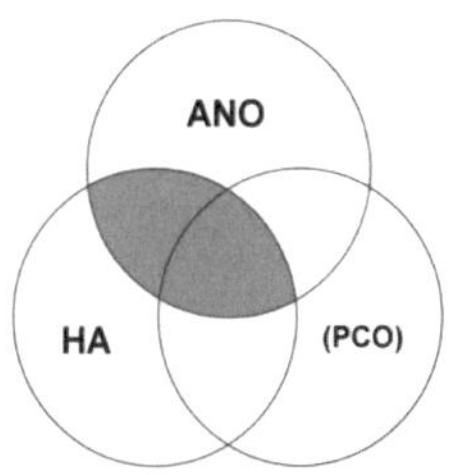

Fig. 3. Visual representation of the patient population diagnosed using the NIH criteria

The size of the circles in Fig. 1, 2, and 3 is arbitrary. The prevalence of HA and ANO in the fertile female population is not known. Around 30% have polycystic ovaries but only a fraction suffers from PCOS (depending on the criteria used for the diagnosis).

The prevalence of PCOS in a community sample of 728 women was found as follows: NIH criteria, 8.7%; AES criteria, 12%, Rotterdam criteria, 17.8% (March et al., 2010). The study used interviews of women who were born in a certain area. The article also emphasizes that at least two third of the cases were previously undiagnosed.

3. PCOS patients in a medical outpatient practice

I work as a private medical practitioner in the Republic of Cyprus on an island in the Eastern Mediterranean; a member state of the EU; with almost exclusively Europid (white, "Caucasian") population. Beyond doing general medicine I am a specialist for endocrinology, diabetes, and metabolic diseases. Private practitioners in Cyprus work independently from the governmental health services, free of territorial or insurance company obligations.

Such practice experience may not be representative for the whole Cypriot population but there have been no published PCOS related data in Cyprus. What we do know is that the prevalence of both Type 2 diabetes and the metabolic syndrome is of the highest in Europe therefore one can suspect a relatively high number of patients living in Cyprus suffering from of all kinds of disorders related to insulin resistance including PCOS (Loizou & al., 2006).

3.1 Patient selection and diagnosis

I raise the possibility of PCOS each time when a female patient turns up presenting any symptom which is compatible with the syndrome; independently of her primary complaint. On detection of other symptoms compatible with PCOS during history taking and physical examination, the suspicion is discussed thoroughly with the patient. Upon informed consent, we continue with the formal diagnostic procedure.

Related disorder	Number	%
Subclinical hypothyroidism	45	61.6
Thyrotoxicosis	3	4.1
Multinodular euthyroidic goitre	10	7.3
De Quervain thyroiditis	1	1.4
Late-onset adrenocortical hyperplasia	3	4.1
Microprolactinoma	3	4.1
Impaired fasting glucose	3	4.1
Impaired glucose tolerance	1	1.4
Type 2 diabetes mellitus	1	1.4
Type 1 diabetes mellitus	1	1.4
Metabolic syndrome	1	1.4
HAIRAN syndrome	1	1.4
Total	73	100

Table 1. The distribution of related disorders co-existing with PCOS in 73 patients

Since 2003, 323 women who had not been using hormonal contraceptives for at least six months have undergone the full diagnostic procedure. The necessary hormonal tests and pelvic ultrasound were performed as recommended by the Rotterdam criteria; occasionally further tests became necessary for differentiation from related disorders. A formal 75 g oral glucose tolerance test was performed in all women diagnosed positively for PCOS except those with known diabetes.

Late-onset adrenocortical hyperplasia was found in one patient and the HAIR-AN syndrome (Hyperandrogenism - Insulin Resistance - Acanthosis Nigricans) in another one without PCOS.

321 women were diagnosed positively for PCOS using the Rotterdam criteria; aging 14 - 46 years (mean 25 years). Only 2 women had no hyperandrogenic signs therefore 319 women (>99%) met also the AES criteria; and only 180 (56%) could have been diagnosed by the NIH criteria.

In 73 patients (22.7%) PCOS was a secondary diagnosis where after the satisfactory control of any related disorder the Rotterdam criteria still applied. The distribution of co-existing disorders of these 73 patients is shown in Table 1.

3.2 Initial symptoms

The following definitions, grading of symptom severity, and abbreviations will be used in this and consecutive sections:

- Acne score: The Global Acne Grading System (Doshi et al., 1997) for its simplicity; requiring only visual assessment of signs in six body areas.
- Hirsutism: Score higher than 8 in the classical Ferriman-Gallwey scale (Ferriman, 1962, as cited in Rosenfield, 1990); by visual assessment of hairiness in nine body areas.
- Weight surplus: body mass index (BMI) ≥25 kg/m^2
  - Overweight: BMI between 25 and 29.9 kg/m^2
  - Obese: BMI between 30 and 34.9 kg/m^2
  - Grossly obese: BMI over 35 kg/m^2
- Abdominal obesity: Waist-to-hip circumference ratio (W/H) ≥0.80
- Irregular menses: menstrual periods <9/year; or periods shorter than 21 or longer than 35 days
- Infertility: no spontaneous pregnancy despite active, non-protected sexual life for at least two years
- Early pregnancy loss (EPL): spontaneous abortion during the first trimester.

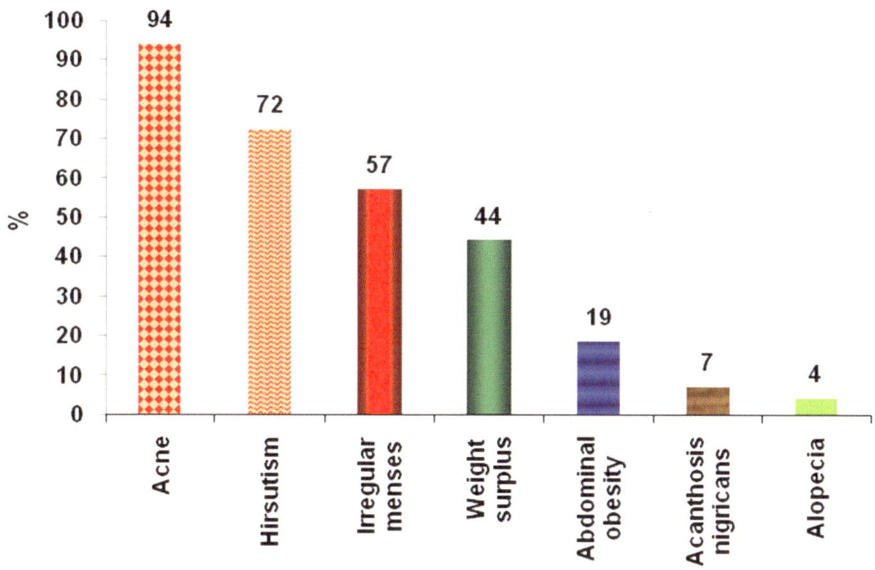

Fig. 4. The distribution of symptoms in 321 women with PCOS at time of diagnosis

The distribution of the initial symptoms of the 321 women found with PCOS according to the Rotterdam criteria (including those with co-existing disorders after full control) is shown in Fig. 4.

The overall majority had easily detectable acne and/or hirsutism with or without laboratory hyperandrogenism; only three patients (0.93%) had laboratory hyperandrogenism without acne or hirsutism. 57% had irregular menstrual periods. 44.3% had weight surplus in the following proportions: overweight, 21.5%; obese, 10.6%; and grossly obese, 12.1%. Acanthosis nigricans occurred only in obese or grossly obese patients.

The fertility rate cannot be verified for the whole group because the majority had not planned pregnancy. Infertility was revealed by history taking in 23 of 108 married women (21.3%); 5 had early pregnancy losses (4.6%). 11 early pregnancy losses occurred in 11 of 85 women (12.9%) having had live births from earlier pregnancies.

4. Testing the efficacy of treatment forms

The following symbols will be used for statistical analysis in this section:

- ***: P<0.001
- ** : P<0.01
- * : P<0.05
- n.s.: not significant

The other symbols and abbreviations are as described in Section 3.2.

4.1 Choice between taking the contraceptive pill or metformin

Before 2002 the standard treatment advice for my patients was the anti-androgenic combined contraceptive pill as mentioned in the introduction. The pill was stopped when the woman wanted to become pregnant; usually the previous symptoms recurred while waiting for (in many cases, only hoping for) conception.

Between 2002 and 2006 I offered the insulin sensitizer metformin treatment to all freshly diagnosed PCOS patients who had contraindications or negative experience with the pill, or simply did not want to take hormonally active medication, or wanted to become pregnant. The efficacy of the two treatment forms (the pill or metformin) was compared in those who completed twelve moths' treatment. The two groups were comparable in size and age distribution. Table 2 shows the results.

	Pill	**Metformin**
Number of patients	17	19
Age (year)	24 (20-31)	23 (15-36)
Acne score	16.9 ± 7.1 - 2.7±2.9 ***	19.7 ± 11.2 - 6.6 ± 6.9 ***
F-G score	15.2 ± 2.7 - 6.6 ± 3.5 ***	16.4 ± 7.2 - 10.9 ± 6.0 ***
BMI	24.0 ± 6.4 - 23.7 ± 5.8 n.s.	26.7 ± 7.8 - 25.4 ± 7.8 n.s.
W/H ratio	0.73 ± 0.1 - 0.71±0.1 n.s.	0.75 ± 0.1 - 0.74 ± 0.1 n.s.

Table 2. Changes during a twelve-month treatment period on the pill or metformin

Both the acne and hirsutism scores decreased significantly during the twelve-month treatment period; BMI and W/H did not change significantly in either group. Further statistical analysis was not made since the two groups differed in the indication of treatment; and the metformin group had more severe symptoms in average. However, this study convinced me that metformin was a simple, safe; and effective first choice of medical treatment in PCOS. In many patients metformin restored the regularity of the menstrual cycles. Spontaneous pregnancies with live births also occurred (Petrányi, 2005; Petrányi & Zaoura, 2007).

4.2 Metformin treatment with or without lifestyle changes

Since 2006 lifestyle changes (Tang & al., 2006) have been advised parallel to the pharmacological treatment for all new patients: the increase of daily physical activity and low glycaemic index diet; including calorie restriction to the overweight. The two treatment forms (metformin with or without lifestyle changes) were compared in the following way (Petrányi & Zaoura, 2011).

Patients from the metformin monotherapy era served as historical control group consisting of 29 women (age 18 to 39 y, mean, 26) to whom the recent metformin + lifestyle changes group was compared consisting of 34 patients with comparable age distribution. The following parameters were recorded every three months during the 6-month observation period: acne and hirsutism scores, body mass index (BMI), waist-to-hip ratio (WH), and the regularity of the menstrual periods. Patients with carbohydrate metabolic disorders (impaired fasting glucose, impaired glucose tolerance, diabetes mellitus) or those who became pregnant during the six-month period were not included in the evaluation.

Table 3 shows the changes of the four easily measurable symptoms during the six-month observation period by the mean ± SD, and the difference (Δ) both in the metformin and the metformin + lifestyle treatment groups; and the difference between the two treatment forms. Not all patients suffered from acne or hirsutism; their number within the groups is also included in the table.

	Metformin (n=29)	**Metformin +lifestyle (n=34)**	**Difference**
Acne	(n=27)	(n=32)	
	20.3±9.9 – 12.4±8.9	25.2±8.2 – 15.9±7.7	
	Δ=7.9 ***	Δ=9.3 ***	1.4 n.s.
Hirsutism	(n=22)	(n=21)	
	15.1±6.0 – 12.8±6.2	11.7±2.1 - 9.2±2.7	
	Δ=2.3 ***	Δ=2.5 ***	0.2 n.s.
BMI	26.6±6.9 - 26.4±6.7	27.5±7 - 26.7±6.3	
	Δ=0.26 n.s.	Δ=0.88 ***	0.62 *
W/H	0.74±0.07 - 0.74±0.07	0.76±0.08 - 0.74±0.07	
	Δ=0.001 n.s.	Δ=0.019 **	0.017 *

Table 3. Comparison of the efficacy of metformin versus metformin + lifestyle treatment

Acne and hirsutism score improved significantly and similarly in both treatment forms.

BMI did not show significant change during the metformin monotherapy but it improved significantly in the combined therapy group. The combined therapy diminished BMI in the overweight women by 1.1 kg/m^2 *** and 0.64 kg/m^2 * in those of normal weight; without causing problem to them.

W/H did not change during metformin monotherapy but decreased significantly with metformin + lifestyle changes.

Table 4 shows the changes in the regularity of menstrual cycles during the six-month treatment period. The proportion of patients who changed from irregular to regular was not significantly different between treatment forms (Fisher's exact test, P=0.29).

	Metformin (n = 29)	**Metformin + lifestyle (n = 34)**
Irregular menses at start	12	22
Remained irregular	4	8
Became regular	8	14
Regular menses at start	17	12
Remained regular	17	12
Became irregular	0	0

Table 4. Number of patients changed regularity of the menstrual cycle during six months

The individual changes in the acne and the hirsutism scores during the combined therapy are shown in the following two figures. The acne score improved in all patients by three months with further improvement by six months (Fig. 5). The hirsutism score did not improve in few patients by three months but everybody improved by six months (Fig. 6).

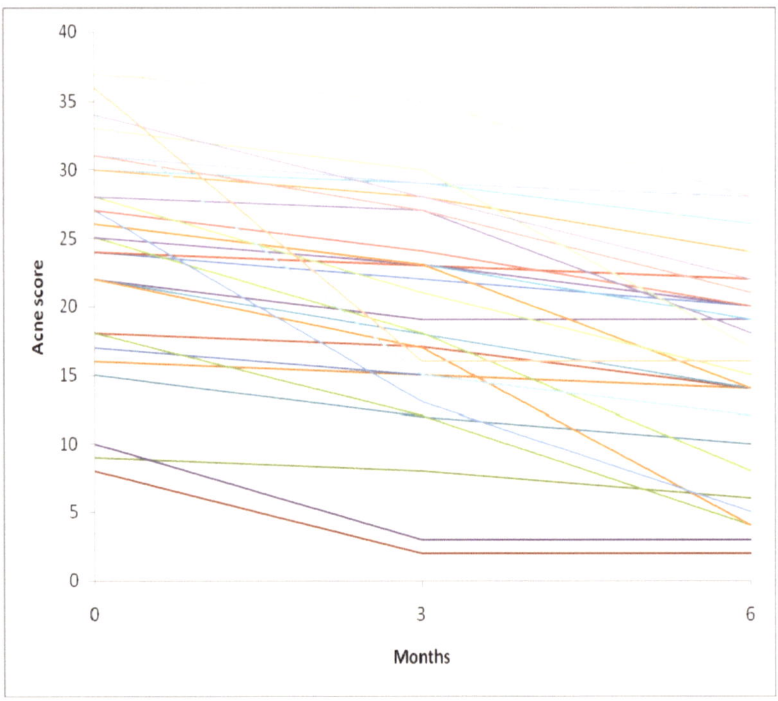

Fig. 5. Individual changes of the acne score under metformin + lifestyle treatment

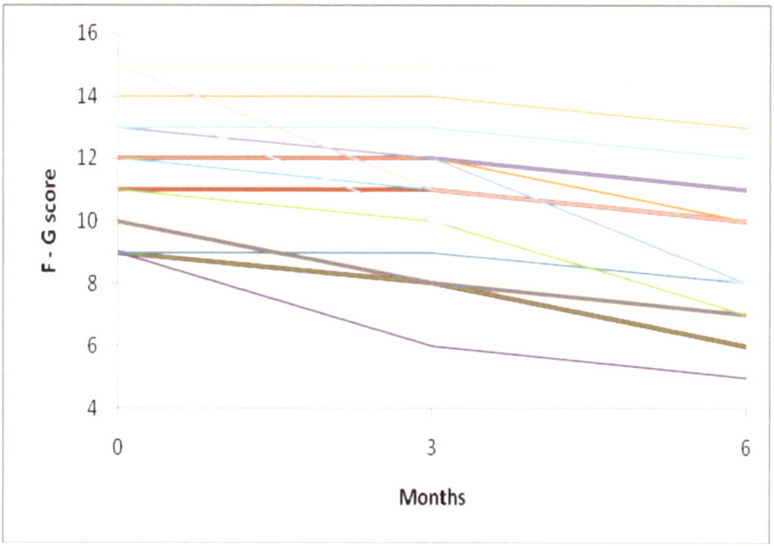

Fig. 6. Individual changes of the hirsutism score under metformin + lifestyle treatment

The favourable change in the body size indexes (BMI and W/H) has been the significant difference between the two treatment forms. In conclusion, the combined treatment can be regarded as superior to metformin monotherapy and therefore I have been offering this combined treatment (under the name of triple basal treatment) for all newly diagnosed patients and for long term use.

4.3 Additional treatment experience with metformin in PCOS

4.3.1 Recurrence of symptoms when treatment is stopped

Whatever treatment option is used its efficacy is limited; stopping treatment results in the renewal of the symptoms. It is most obvious for treatment approaches which have nothing to do with the pathophysiology of PCOS like hair removal, dermatological treatment for acne (local agents, antibiotics, and isotretinoin). After stopping the contraceptive pill, symptoms usually come back within a few months. This applies also to lifestyle changes and/or metformin.

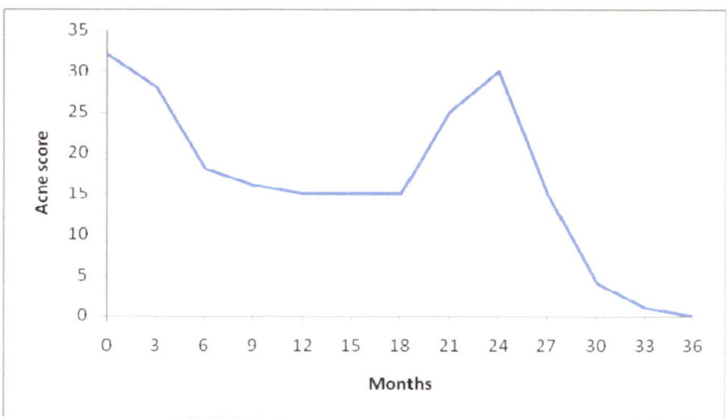

Fig. 7. Relapse of acne on stopping metformin; improvement on treatment restart

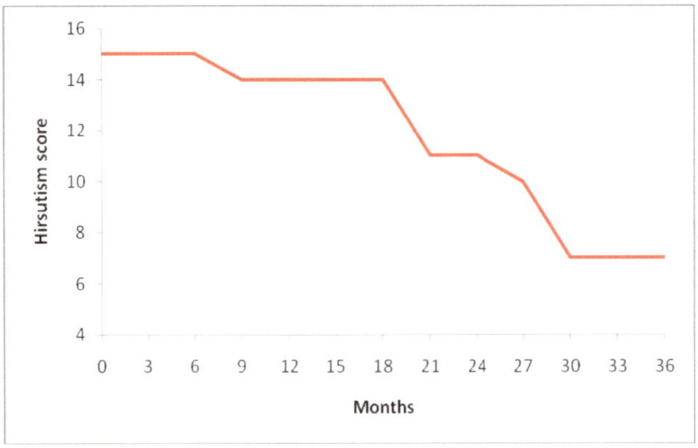

Fig. 8. Stagnation of hirsutism on stopping metformin; improvement on treatment restart

Fig. 7 and Fig. 8 show this happen in a patient who initially was responding favourably to long-term metformin treatment. After a while the improvement became unsatisfactory and by 21 months acne relapsed; by 24 months hirsutism stagnated. Then she acknowledged that she had stopped metformin taking months before. On restart of metformin both symptoms improved and one year later she was free from acne and hirsutism.

This case demonstrates that acne responds to metformin treatment within three months and worsens within three months after stopping treatment. The effect on hirsutism takes more months to show; and the beneficial effect still lasts for more months after stopping treatment.

This was not the only case of non-compliance with long-term treatment recommendations. More difficult to maintain is the adherence to lifestyle changes; especially the achievement of slimming in the overweight; like in other metabolic disturbances.

4.3.2 Improvement of fertility

Ten previously infertile women expressed the desire for having a baby before the initiation of metformin treatment. Metformin taking during pregnancy and breast feeding were discussed and encouraged; all consented.

Eleven conceptions happened among nine women while taking metformin; notably varying between the first and 29th month of treatment; the majority (seven conceptions) occurred after the 6th month of treatment. No gestational diabetes or other complications occurred during pregnancy. Two pregnancies ended with early loss. Nine healthy and normal weight babies were born in term and were breast fed for at least three months. All children showed normal development.

4.3.3 No recurrence of preeclampsia during the next pregnancy when taking metformin

One woman had five previous pregnancies with preeclampsia; one pregnancy was terminated because of the serious condition and one pregnancy was lost early. She presented with thyrotoxicosis caused by toxic multinodular goitre but PCOS could be diagnosed after thyroidectomy and stabilisation with levothyroxine. She conceived during the first month of taking metformin and she continued metformin throughout this pregnancy upon my advice. Preeclampsia did not recur during this pregnancy and a healthy baby was born in term (Petrányi, 2005).

5. Discussion

I have seen many, mostly young women suffering from PCOS. Despite growing interest by the medical public and remarkable progress in research during the past two decades, the medical literature has not provided equivocal help how to treat PCOS. It is true that there is no evidence based universal treatment option but the advice found in textbooks, consensus statements and "experts' opinions" does not give clear guidance what to do in general with these patients. The treatment advice is usually grouped around the symptoms of PCOS but not against PCOS as a pathophysiological entity, which is a chronic, progressive disorder leading to irreversible damage through late complications.

Most publications deal with the fertility aspects of PCOS regardless of the other endocrine and metabolic aspects of the disease. Infertility is an just once important issue but does not affect all women with PCOS and even so only for a limited period while the other problems exist and cause harm throughout their life. Usually fertility studies are limited to six months - the time length beyond clomiphene stimulation (the advocated treatment of choice for PCOS related infertility) cannot be recommended (BNF 2010). Such studies are unsuitable to demonstrate whether other but longer treatment forms could not result in similar or better outcome and safety records (avoiding overstimulation, ensuring singleton pregnancies, prevention of macrosomia, gestational diabetes, preeclampsia etc). Longer treatment would of course require more patience from the patient but could give more chance to improve other pathological processes in favour of the general health of the woman. Fertility results are especially disappointing in obese women; they have only a 1:4 chance to give live birth using clomiphene stimulation (Legro et al., 2007). Assisted reproduction methods are complicated, very costly; and increase the risk of malformations (El-Chaar et al., 2009).

The majority of my patients have been suffering from disturbing symptoms of hyperandrogenism (almost all from acne and/or hirsutism, rarely from alopecia); and the metabolic consequences of insulin resistance (obesity, abdominal obesity). Irregular menses is also frequent among them but it is rarely the main complaint. Few in my clientele wanted to be pregnant urgently. According to my medical judgement these women need a long-term, uniform treatment (knowing that short-term attempts are unsuitable) which is simple, cheap, safe, effective for almost all features of PCOS, and can be combined with other treatment forms if the improvement is not satisfactory in certain symptoms.

Whatever is the main complaint of the patient, we will certainly find a long list of symptoms during the diagnostic procedure. Some of these are pre-requisites of the diagnosis like hyperandrogenism (that rarely exists without somatic signs); anovulation related symptoms (oligo-amenorrhoea, sub- or infertility); and the well-known metabolic consequences of PCOS cannot be left out: weight surplus that can be extreme, carbohydrate metabolic problems, lipid disorders - all these deserve treatment and/or preventive measures not to develop into late cardiovascular problems. We should also think of the increased dangers during pregnancy of PCOS patients: pregnancy loss, gestational diabetes, macrosomia. These all should be discussed with the patient before offering any treatment.

My observations with metformin in PCOS proved to meet these requirements, and the combination with lifestyle changes helped also the weight problems, too. I cannot use placebo control; the patients come for effective treatment not for experimenting.

It is not only my opinion that PCOS should be dealt with like any other chronic metabolic disorders (diabetes, obesity or the metabolic syndrome), which all have insulin resistance in the background and end up with similar late complications. We have to think about the future of the patient, not only the actual complaints.

Insulin resistance is hypothesised in the background of PCOS even if there is no simple and precise method to prove it individually. Fortunately, the measurement of insulin during the oral glucose tolerance test is not included in the recommendations of the diagnostic procedure; this imprecise method may be used only for statistical comparisons of different populations or treatment forms. Treatments which increase insulin sensitivity have been proved useful in PCOS for all aspects of the disease. Reduction of obesity, increased physical activity (lifestyle changes), and insulin sensitizers - primarily, metformin has been found effective in treating PCOS. Other insulin sensitizers have also been tested but because of their controversy in diabetes and unknown safety in pregnancy they cannot be recommended in PCOS for the time being.

Metformin is not a miracle drug but it is cheap and safe, it can be administered without time limitation; and has very few contraindications in the relatively young and (in this respect) healthy female population suffering from PCOS. Its long-term and lasting metabolic benefits are well known from more than fifty years' clinical experience in diabetes and beyond; and can be used from the age of ten onwards (Bailey et al., 2007).

Metformin has not been licensed for PCOS in any country in the world. This prevents or restricts its prescription for PCOS in some countries. The patients' acceptance of metformin is overwhelming (Hillary et al., 2009); researchers complain that patients do not want to cease treatment, even for few months because they considered the treatment as effective (Muth at al., 2004).

Some patients experience gastrointestinal disturbance (bloating, abdominal pain, watery diarrhoea) or sometimes nausea, metallic taste while taking metformin. This can be avoided in the majority of cases by gradual dose increase. Only few patients cannot tolerate even one 500 mg tablet daily. I have no personal experience with the extended release formulation or the powdered form, which have been developed to overcome these unpleasant symptoms.

One side effect deserves real consideration: metformin may cause or exaggerate vitamin B_{12} deficiency; therefore annual test for B_{12} level is advisable for long-term metformin users to select who needs vitamin B_{12} supplementation.

Treatment experience with metformin in PCOS comes from relatively short studies but longer ones has also been published (Cheang et al., 2009, Oppelt et al., 2010). Detailed discussion in favour of the use, including long-term use of metformin in PCOS for all possible aspects, indications, contraindications, and safety issues has also been published in growing numbers (Diamanti-Kandarakis et al., 2010; Nestler, 2008; Palomba et al., 2009) including metformin taking during pregnancy and lactation.

Vitamin D is probably the next candidate substance to be used widely in PCOS especially in the obese patients (Kosta et al., 2009). The high prevalence of depression in patients with PCOS (Dokras et al., 2011) also requires true consideration but these topics are not discussed in this chapter.

6. Conclusions

The patients want (and deserve) effective treatment. There is no evidence based general treatment option for all patients suffering from PCOS but the advice to treat the patients according to their main complaint (or symptomatically) is also not evidence based.

We'd better do our best using common sense; based on available evidence combined with our experience to provide benefit (Stuebe, 2011).

For the time being the combination of lifestyle changes and metformin treatment appears to be beneficial for the majority of patients suffering from PCOS by controlling their symptoms with potentials for preventing progression and most complications.

Until a sound and better solution is found, my medical advice to all newly diagnosed patients with PCOS from the time of diagnosis (even from puberty) is this:

- The patient diagnosed with PCOS should be fully informed about her medical condition; which of her symptoms are connected to this disorder, and what other ill conditions may develop by time.
- The patient should know that at present there is no final cure for the problem but a long-term, cheap and safe treatment combination may revert or attenuate most of the symptoms.
- The initial treatment (triple basal treatment) consists of long-term lifestyle changes: the increase of the daily physical activity and a low glycaemic index diet (with calorie restriction for the overweight to normalize body weight) and taking metformin tablets.
- Metformin should be started stepwise. The starting dose is one 500 mg tablet after dinner; increased to twice daily (after breakfast - after dinner) after one week and to three times daily (after breakfast, after lunch and after dinner) from the third week onwards. Eventual side-effects must be consulted with the doctor; any dose increase should be postponed until the dissolution of the disturbing phenomena.
- If certain symptoms do not improve satisfactorily in suitable time (depending on the nature of the symptom; for example, acne in six months, and hirsutism in one year; stagnation of weight surplus; oligo-amenorrhoea continues, infertility) the following options should be considered:
  - Revision of diagnosis
  - Compliance with treatment recommendations
  - Further calorie restriction in the overweight with or without increased dose of metformin (up to daily 2000-2500 mg)
  - Addition of other medication depending on the nature of the problem:

    - Anti-androgenic contraceptives, spironolactone, flutamide
    - Dermatological treatment for acne (antibiotics, isotretinoin)
    - Ovarian stimulation and/or other fertility interventions upon consultation with the fertility specialist.
- The triple basal treatment may help the patient conceive. Effective contraceptive methods should be discussed with all those who do not want become pregnant or take teratogenic medication (anti-androgens, isotretinoin) before commencing treatment.
- The patient should be reviewed for symptoms and adherence to the therapeutic advice every three months for at least one year and thereafter at least twice yearly if the condition improves satisfactorily.
- Annual monitoring of kidney and liver function, lipid profile, glycosylated haemoglobin, vitamin B_{12} levels is mandatory.

This proposal remains a working hypothesis until properly planned, long-term clinical studies find a better alternative.

7. References

Azziz, R., Carmina, E., Dewailly, D., Diamanti-Kandarakis, E., Escobar-Morreale, H.F., Futterweit, W., Janssen, O.E., Legro, R.S., Norman, R.J., Taylor, A.E. & Witchel, S. (2009). The Androgen Excess and PCOS Society criteria for the polycystic ovary syndrome: the complete task force report. *Fertility and Sterility,* Vol.91, No.2, (February 2009), pp. 456-488, ISSN 1556-5653

Azziz, R., Woods, K. S., Reyna, R., Key, T.J., Knochenhauer, E.S. & Yildiz, B.O. (2004). The prevalence and features of the polycystic ovary syndrome in an unselected population. *Journal of Clinical Endocrinology and Metabolism,* Vol.89, No.6, (June 2004), pp. 2745-2749, ISSN 1945-7197

Bailey, C.J., Campbell, I.W., Chan, J.C.N., Davidson, J.A., Howlett, H.C.S., Ritz, P (Eds). (2007). *Metformin – The gold standard.* Wiley & Sons Ltd, ISBN 978-0-470-72644-2, Chichester

BNF 2010. *British National Formulary,* Vol. 60 (September 2010) BMJ Group & Pharmaceutical Press, ISBN 978-0-85369-931-6, London, p. 453

Cheang, K.I., Huszar, J.M., Best, A.M., Sharma, S., Essah, P.A. & Nestler, J.E. (2009).Long-term effect of metformin on metabolic parameters in the polycystic ovary syndrome. *Diabetes & Vascular Disease Research,* Vol. 6, No.2, (April 2009), pp. 110-119, ISSN 1752-8984

Diamanti-Kandarakis, E., Christakou, C.D., Kandaraki, E. & Economou, F.N. (2010). Metformin: an old medication of new fashion: evolving new molecular mechanisms and clinical implications in polycystic ovary syndrome. *European Journal of Endocrinology* Vol. 162, No.2, (February 2010), pp. 193–212, ISSN 0804-4643

Dokras, A., Clifton, S., Futterweit, W. & Wild, R. (2011). Increased risk for abnormal depression scores in women with polycystic ovary syndrome: a systematic review. *Obstetrics and Gynecology,* Vol. 117, No.1 (January 2011), pp. 145-152 ISSN 1873-233x

Doshi, A., Zaheer, A. & Stiller, M. (1997) A comparison of current acne grading systems and proposal of a novel system. *International Journal of Dermatology,* Vol.36, No.6, (June 1997), pp. 416-418, ISSN 1365-4632

El-Chaar, D., Yang, Q., Gao, J, Bottomley, J., Leader, A., Wen S.W. & Walker, M. (2009). Risk of birth defects increased in pregnancies conceived by assisted reproduction. *Fertility and Sterility*, Vol.92, No.5, (November 2009), pp. 1557-1561, ISSN1556-5653

Hillary, C., Conway, A., Waung, J., Levy, M & Howlett, T. (2009). Patient reported outcomes for the use of metformin in polycystic ovarian syndrome (PCOS). *Endocrine Abstracts*, Vol.19 (March 2010), P296, Congress of the British Endocrine Societies, ISSN 1479-6848, Harrogate, March 2009

Kosta, K., Yavropoulou, M.P., Anastasiou, O. & Yovos, G. (2009). Role of vitamin D treatment in glucose metabolism in polycystic ovary syndrome. *Fertility and Sterility*, Vol.92, No.3, (September 2009), pp. 1053-1058, ISSN 1556-5653

Legro, R. S., Barnhart, H.X., Schlaff, W.D., Carr, B.R., Diamond, M.P., Carson, S.A., Steinkampf, M.P., Coutifaris, C., McGovern, P.G., Cataldo, N.A., Gosman, G.C., Nestler, J.E., Giudice, C., Leppert, P.C., & Myers, E.R. (2007). Clomiphene, metformin, or both for infertility in the polycystic ovary syndrome. *New England Journal of Medicine*, Vol.356, No. 6, (February 2007), pp. 551-566, ISSN 1533-4406

Loizou, T., Pouloukas, S., Tountas, C, Thanopoulou, A. & Karamanos, V. (2006). An epidemiologic study on the prevalence of diabetes, glucose intolerance, and metabolic syndrome in the adult population of the Republic of Cyprus. *Diabetes Care*, Vol. 29, No.7, (July 2006), 1714-1715, ISSN 0149-5992

Mani, H., Levy, M., Howlett, T., Gray, L., Webb, D., Srinivasan, B, Khnuti, K. & Davies, M. (2010). Apparent under-reporting of polycystic ovary syndrome in primary care. *Endocrine Abstracts*, Vol.21 (March 2010), P324, Congress of the British Endocrine Societies, ISSN 1479-6848, Manchester, March 2010

March, W.A.; Moore, V.M., Willson, K.J., Phillips, D.I.W., Norman, R.J. & Davies, M.J. (2010). The prevalence of polycystic ovary syndrome in a community sample assessed under contrasting diagnostic criteria. *Human Reproduction*, Vol.25, No.2, (February 2010), pp. 544-551, ISSN 1460-2350

Muth, S., Norman, J., Sattar, N. & Fleming, R. (2004). Women with polycystic ovary syndrome (PCOS) often undergo protracted treatment with metformin and are disinclined to stop: indications for a change in licensing arrangements? *Human Reproduction*, Vol. 19, No.12, (December 2004), 1460-2350, ISSN 1460-2350

Nestler, J.E. (2008). Metformin for the treatment of the polycystic ovary syndrome. *New England Journal of Medicine*, Vol.358, No. 1, (January 2007), pp. 47-54, ISSN 1533-4406

Oppelt, P. G., Mueller, A., Jentsch, K., D., Kronawitter, D., Reissmann, C., Dittrich, R., Beckmann, M.W. & Cupisti, S. (2010) The effect of metformin treatment for 2 years without caloric restriction on endocrine and metabolic parameters in women with polycystic ovary syndrome. *Experimental Clinical Endocrinology and Diabetes*, Vol. 118, No.9, (September 2010), pp. 633-637, ISSN 1439-3646

Palomba, S., Falbo, A., Zullo, F. & Orio, F. (2009) Evidence-based and potential benefits of metformin in the polycystic ovary syndrome: a comprehensive review. *Endocrine Reviews* . Vol. 30, No.1, (January 2009) pp. 1–50, 1945-7189

Pasquali, R., Stener-Victorin, E., Yildiz, B.O., Duleba, A.J., Hoeger, K., Mason, H., Homburg, R., Hickey, T., Franks, S., Tapanainen, J.S., Balen, A., Abbott, D.H., Diamanti-Kandarakis, E. & Legro, R.S. (2011). Research in polycystic ovary syndrome today and tomorrow. *Clinical Endocrinology,* Vol.74, No.4, (April 2011), pp. 424-433, ISSN 0300-0664

Petrányi, G. (2005). Treatment experience with metformin in polycystic ovary syndrome [in Hungarian with English abstract]. *Orvosi Hetilap,* Vol.146, No.21, (May 2005), pp. 1151-1155, ISSN 1788-6120

Petrányi, G. & Zaoura, M. (2007). Five-year experience with metformin in polycystic ovary syndrome. *Endocrine Abstracts,* Vol.14 (2007), P493, 9th European Congress of Endocrinology, ISSN 1479-6848 (online). Budapest, April 2007

Petrányi, G. & Zaoura, M. (2011). Metformin treatment with or without life style changes in the polycystic ovary syndrome. *Endocrine Abstracts,* Vol.26 (April 2011), P93, 13th European Congress of Endocrinology, ISSN 1479-6848, Rotterdam, April 2011

Rosenfield, R.L. (1990). Hyperandrogenism in peripubertal girls. *Pediatric Clinics of North America,* Vol.37, No.6 (June 1990), pp. 1333-1346, ISSN 0031-3955

Stuebe, A.M. (2011). Level IV evidence - Adverse anecdote and clinical practice. . *New England Journal of Medicine,* Vol.365, No. 1, (July 2011), pp.8-9, ISSN 1533-4406

Tang, T., Glanville,J., Hayden, C., White, D., Barth, J.H. & Balen, A.H. (2006). Combined lifestyle modification and metformin in obese patients with polycystic ovary syndrome. A randomized, placebo-controlled, double-blind multicentre study. *Human Reproduction,* Vol.21, No.1 (January 2006), pp. 80-89, ISSN 1460-2350

The Rotterdam ESHRE/ASRM-sponsored PCOS consensus workshop group. (2004). Revised 2003 consensus on diagnostic criteria and long-term health risks related to polycystic ovary syndrome (PCOS), *Fertility and Sterility,* Vol. 81, No.1 (January 2004), pp. 41-47, ISSN 1556-5653

Wilson, J.F. (2011). In the Clinic: The Polycystic ovary Syndrome, *Annals of Internal Medicine,* Vol. 154, No. 3, (February 2011), pp. 1-14, ISSN 1539-3704

9

Implications of Insulin Resistance / Hyperinsulinemia on Reproductive Function in Infertile Women with Polycystic Ovary Syndrome

Tetsurou Sakumoto[1,3], Yoshimitsu Tokunaga[1], Yoko Terada[1], Hideaki Tanaka[2], Makoto Nohara[3], Aritoshi Nakaza[3] and Masahiro Higashi[3]

[1]*Alba Okinawa Clinic*

[2]*Tanaka Clinic*

[3] *The Department of Infertility and Endocrinology, Tomishiro Central Hospital*

Japan

1. Introduction

One of the most common reproductive endocrine diseases that impact many young women worldwide is polycystic ovary syndrome (PCOS). This hormonal problem affects 4 - 18% of women of reproductive age exhibiting various symptoms, such as irregular menstruation, hirsutism, infertility and metabolic disorders (LJ. Moran, et al. 2011). These symptoms in PCOS women are strongly correlated with overweight and obesity. Also, women with PCOS are likely to have metabolic disorders, such as abnormality of glucose and lipid metabolisms that are inevitably involved in diabetes mellitus and coronary artery diseases, respectively (ML. Traub, 2011). Concerning metabolic syndrome in young women, abnormalities in glucose metabolism are seen earlier than dyslipidemia as the initial manifestation; thus, glucose metabolism is suggested to be evaluated first (A. Fulghesu, et al. 2011). Insulin resistance / hyperinsulinemia is frequently associated with 40-50 % of women having PCOS, especially obese women (JE. Nestler, et al. 2002). Furthermore, obese women with PCOS are more likely indicative of insulin resistance than lean women with or without PCOS (P. Acien, et al. 1999). It is well-known that insulin resistance manifests in glucose tolerance test (GTT) prior to diabetes mellitus and coronary artery diseases (ML. Traub, 2011). Based on the recent reports, insulin resistance / hyperinsulinemia correlates with implantation disturbances and causes infertility in PCOS women (DJ, Jakubowicz, et al. 2001). Also, it is reported that the rate of early pregnancy loss is higher in women with PCOS than in normal women (DJ. Jakubowicz, et al. 2002). Thereby, insulin resistance / hyperinsulinemia is strongly linked to women with PCOS and this correlation has to be studied in details. As for obesity and overweight, which also strongly relates with PCOS, body mass index (BMI) is suggested to contribute to severity while assessing many problems, such as miscarriage, anovulation, infertility and increased prevalence of diabetes mellitus (JX. Wang et al. 2002; RJ. Norman, et al. 2002). Also, weight reduction is effective to improve the PCOS symptoms in obese and overweight infertile women, and insulin sensitizing drug, such as metformin, ameliorates menstrual cycle and ovulation in PCOS women (J. Vrbikova, et al. 2002; B. Baysal, et al. 2001; R. Fleming, et al. 2002). From the above-mentioned facts, the adverse effects of insulin resistance / hyperinsulinemia are inextricable with infertile women with PCOS and cause ovulatory disturbance, implantation failure and early pregnancy loss (in early stage). Yet, the lifestyle changes, such as weight reduction and dietary modification, as well as the use of insulin sensitizing agents are crucial for the improvement of reproductive functions for PCOS women.

2. Insulin resistance / hyperinsulinemia and PCOS

The diagnostic criteria for PCOS followed in most of the studies are in accordance with Rotterdam PCOS consensus 2003 (BCJM. Fauser, 2003). Insulin resistance affects 70% of PCOS women, while 10% have diabetes mellitus (DM) (R. Freeman, et al. 2010; K. Farrell, et al. 2010; F. Ovalle, et al. 2002). Over three years, 25% of PCOS women with normal glucose metabolism can become those with abnormal glucose metabolism (MH. Pesant, et al. 2011). Therefore, glucose level alone has lack of sensitivity to predict metabolic disorders in patients with PCOS. In turn, the assessment of insulin resistance is important to evaluate the metabolic conditions in women with PCOS.

Obese women with PCOS are seen more insulin resistant, hyperandrogenic and hypertriglyceridemic although insulin and metabolic indices tend to be similar in lean type of women with PCOS and those without PCOS (P. Acien, et al. 1999). Reproductive disorders in patients with PCOS may manifest insulin resistance. Irregularity of menstrual cycle has been correlated with insulin resistance (T. Strowitzki, et al. 2010). It is reported that hyperinsulinemia in PCOS patients with lower pregnancy implantation rate may be reflected in the local endometrial level due to impairment of insulin receptor action (R. Fornes, et al. 2010). Also, high concentration of insulin in follicular fluid might lead to low pregnancy outcomes in patients with PCOS after in vitro fertilization (S. Takikawa, et al. 2010). Although many areas of PCOS have not been fully understood yet, insulin resistance / hyperinsulinemia plays an important role of pathogenesis and pathophysiology in PCOS.

3. Assessment of Insulin resistance / hyperinsulinemia

In order to assess insulin resistance / hyperinsulinemia, the relationship between insulin sensitivity and insulin secretion is needed to be understood despite their complicated interaction (C. Cobeli, et al. 2007). In general, up-regulation of insulin secretion corresponds to the reduction in insulin sensitivity for healthy subjects with normal glucose tolerance (K. Færch, et al. 2010). Thus, insulin sensitivity and insulin secretion are inversely related to each other and can be seen in a hyperbolic manner. These two variables constantly appear in human with the same levels of glucose tolerance, known as the disposition index (K. Faerch, et al. 2010). The assessment of the disposition index can be calculated from the measurement of insulin sensitivity and insulin secretion by the euglycaemic-hyperinsulinemic clamp technique in combination with the intravenous glucose tolerance test (MA. Adbul-Ghani, et al. 2006a; K. Færch, et al. 2008; M. Laakso et al. 2008). Additionally, a hepatic insulin resistance can be estimated the following multiplication:

1 / (endogenous glucose production x basal insulin concentration)
(C. Brøns et al. 2009; AC. Alibegovic et al. 2009).

A low disposition index indicates the increase in insulin secretion meaning the dysfunction of islet beta-cells; then, resulting in an inadequate hyperinsulinemia (B. Ahre´n, et al. 2002).

There is no concrete measurement of insulin resistance universally. However, various types of methods to measure insulin resistance are proposed, such as hyperinsulinemic euglycernic clamp techniques, fasting methods and 75 g of glucose tolerance test (GTT). In our studies, hyperinsulinemic euglycernic clamp techniques are not utilized because it requires intravenous infusions, extensive time and significant financial resources. With combination of fasting methods and 75g of GTT, insulin resistance and hyperinsulinemia are assessed in our studies. As an index of insulin resistance, the homeostasis model assessment ratio (HOMA-R) is calculated by the formula:

HOMA-R = Fasting insulin level (μU/ml) x
Fasting glucose levels (mg/dl) / 405
(DR. Mattews, et al. 1985).

As a result of the assessment for insulin resistance, HOMA-R with greater than 1.6 is determined to be insulin resistance (H. Tanaka, et al. 2005). In addition, the amount of insulin level with greater than 100 μU/ml at any minutes, or 65 μU/ml at 120 minutes is determined to be hyperinsulinemia. HOMA- β estimates steady state of pancreatic β-cell function by the measurement of fasting plasma glucose and insulin concentrations. It is strongly correlated with high concentration of glycemia as a determinant of its degree. The formula is as follows:

HOMA- β (%) = Fasting plasma insulin (μ U/ml) x 360 /
(Fasting plasma glucose (mmol/L) - 63)
(DR. Mattews, et al. 1985).

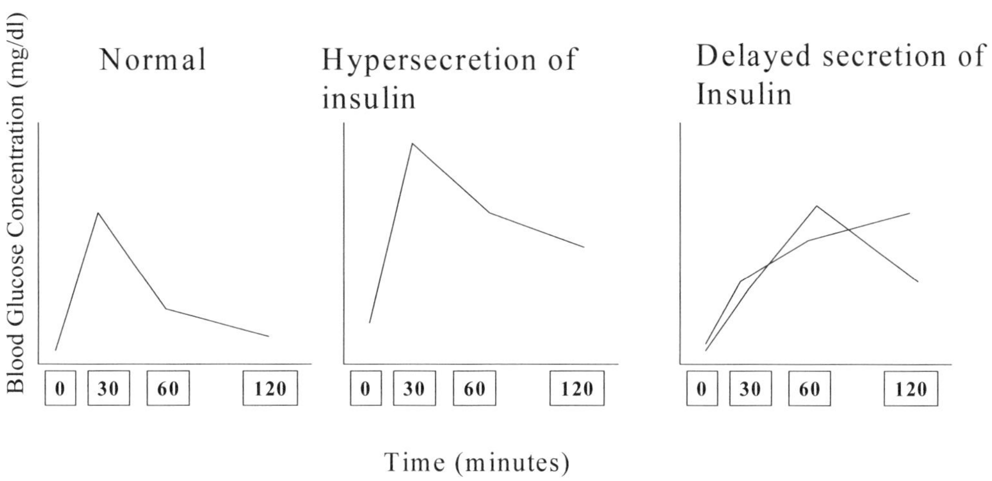

Fig. 1. Assessment of insulin secretion after GTT, showing blood glucose concentration (mg/dl) on Y axes and time (minutes) on X axes.

Therefore, HOMA- β is effective for understanding progressive type 2 DM. Because almost all of the subjects in our study show normal range of glucose levels, HOMA- β is not analyzed.

Seventy-five grams of glucose is used for the patients in GTT and blood samples are collected at 0, 30, 60 and 120 minutes for circulating blood sugar and insulin levels. As shown in Fig. 1, three types of insulin secretions are indicated. In normal type, highest peak of insulin is secreted at 30 min. and gradually decreased. In hypersecretion type, the insulin level indicates high response at any points - i.e. 0, 30, 60, 120 min. compared with normal. In delayed type, the insulin level gradually increases and/or does not return to normal level at 120 min. Both hypersecretion and delayed secretion indicate insulin abnormalities.

4. Insulin resistance / hyperinsulinemia and lifestyle intervention

Lifestyle management may contribute to the improvement of metabolic complication in overweight and obese women with PCOS. It also correlates with reproductive function for triggering ovulation and maintaining pregnancy by modifying lifestyle as necessary (LJ. Moran, et al. 2009). Control in weight for health benefit, instead of weight-loss purpose only, helps all women with PCOS and it improves psychological distress, hyperandrogenemia and menstrual disturbances that are associated with great food cravings (SS. Lim, et al. 2009). In fact, approximately 5 to 10% of weight loss is enough to ameliorate psychological distress, ovulatory dysfunction, and metabolic disorders (C. Galletly, et al. 1996). Modifying both moderate physical activity and dietary management might also support PCOS women to result in clinical benefit. Simple cardio exercises, such as walking for at least 30 min. per day, are beneficial for PCOS women (ET. Poehlman, et al. 2000).

Although there is still more research needed to conclude the advantageous dietary approach for PCOS women, dietary management may be helpful for improving their reproductive and metabolic functions if the strategies are nutritionally balanced and sustainable for them (LJ. Moran, et al. 2009).

From the above-mentioned point of views, the improvement of lifestyle management and its disciplinary approach that encourages PCOS patients to have good physical activities and dietary strategies may be strongly supportive with targeted medical treatment. In other words, medical treatment and lifestyle therapy should be provided in parallel.

5. Insulin resistance / hyperinsulinemia and ovulatory disorders

The presence of hyperandrogenism in lean and obese women with PCOS is strongly correlated with hyperinsulinemia (RJ. Chang, et al. 1983; A. Dunaif, et al. 1987; A. Dunaif, et al. 1989; A. Dunaif, et al. 1992). The hyperandrogenism results from both increased adrenal and ovarian androgen production (DA. Ehrmann, et al. 1995; RL. Rosenfield, et al. 1990; E. Carmina, et al. 1992; DA. Ehrmann, et al. 1992). Insulin acts via its receptor and appears to contribute ovarian and adrenal androgen biosynthesis (RL. Barbieri, et al. 1986; RL. Barbien, et al. 1988), which amplifies luteinizing hormone induced androgen production by the theca cells and results in hyperandrogenemia (R. Nahum, et al. 1995; DS. Willis, et al. 1998). To improve hyperinsulinemia is effective for circulating androgens to decline to normal level (RD. Murray, et al. 2000). In addition, the upregulation of insuin-like grouth factor- I (IGF-I) receptors may be caused from hyperinsulinemia. IGF-I receptors have the potential to stimulate LH-induced androgen synthesis and suppress IGF-binding protein I (IGF-BPI) production by liver (AM. Suikkan, et al. 1988; AM. Suikkan, 1989). Hepatic sex hormone binding globulin (SHBG) production may be inhibited by insulin (N. Botwood, et al. 1995) and it increases the bioactive androgen that eventually causes virilization.

In PCOS, many small antral follicles are characteristically recognized by ultra sonography. These small antral follicles are due to the arrest of growth after reaching a diameter of 5 to 8mm. The arrest of small follicles may be caused by premature activation of LH-mediated terminal differentiation of granulosa cells (S. Franks, et al. 1996). In the normal menstrual cycle, granulosa cells of the dominant follicle become responsive to LH in mid-follicular phase at a follicular diameter of 10mm (SG. Hillier 1994). On the other hand, granulose cells from follicles as small as 4mm in diameter of anovulatory PCOS are responsive to LH. This response to LH is remarkably amplified by insulin. The premature activation of granulosa cells to LH induces terminal differentiation, resulting in the arrest of follicle growth (S. Franks, et al. 1999).

In PCOS patients with ovulatory disorders, insulin resistance, hyperinsulinemia, BMI and visceral fat are studied. As shown in Table 1, values of BMI, HOMA-R and visceral fat accumulation result to be various. However, the results of GTT show abnormal pattern of insulin secretion in most of the cases with PCOS. The effects of treatment with insulin sensitizing agents are present. If ovulation induction with metformin or pioglitazone is failed during one to two cycles, clomiphen citrate is utilized along with one of the insulin sensitizing agents. In PCOS, ten out of 11 cases result in ovulation by treating with insulin sensitizing agents: 5 cases with metformin and 5 cases with pioglitazone. Based on the assessment of GTT including insulin secretion levels, insulin-sensitizing agents are effective for treatment of ovulation induction.

case	BMI	HOMA	obesity with visceral fat	GTT/ insulin secretion pattern	treatment	ovulation
1	19.4	0.68	none	normal	P + CC	positive
2	20.8	1.69	none	delayed	P + CC	positive
3	23.7	0.65	none	delayed	P + CC	positive
4	24.8	2.12	none	delayed	P + CC	positive
5	25.6	1.50	none	normal	P	positive
6	25.8	1.42	none	delayed	M	positive
7	27.3	4.04	present	hypersecrestion	M + CC	negative
8	27.6	1.45	present	diabetes	M	positive
9	27.8	2.50	present	hypersecrestion	M + CC	positive
10	28.0	4.00	none	hypersecrestion	M	positive
11	32.0	3.43	none	hypersecrestion	M	positive

* P = Pioglitazone
M = Metformin
CC= Clomiphene Citrate

Table 1. BMI, HOMA, obesity with visceral fat, insulin secretion after GTT in 11 cases with PCOS, and ovulation results by the treatment of insulin sensitizing agents

6. Insulin resistance / hyperinsulinemia and insulin sensitizing agents in PCOS

As shown in Table 2, insulin-sensitizing agents, metformin and pioglitazone, are most effective on ovulatory disorder in PCOS with insulin resistance and abnormal insulin secretion. It is well known that the functional mechanisms are different in both of the agents. Metformin is an oral biguanide, category B drug for pregnant women, which has been approved for treatment of type 2 diabetes mellitus. It is thought to affect multiple metabolic pathways, decreasing glucose absorption and suppressing hepatic glucose output and gluconeogenesis (F. Mcyer, et al. 1967; N. Wollen, et al 1988). Also metformin directly inhibits androgen production in human thecal cells (GR. Attia, et al. 2001). Side effects are rare, and gastrointestinal disturbances, such as abdominal pain and nausea, rarely cause discontinuation of treatment.

On the other hand, pioglitazone is a thiazolidinedione derivative to be used for treatment of type 2 diabetes mellitus. It is more potent in glucose-lowering effect and favorable effects on abdominal lipid levels including the decrease in circulating triglyceride and free fatty acid levels. Pioglitazone may affect and differentiate on adipocytes via peroxisome proliferator-activated receptorγ (PPARγ). As a result, differentiated adipocytes regulate insulin sensitivity and improve insulin resistance (T Yamauchi, et al. 2001). Side effects are reported as hepatic disturbance and edema but these side effects are tolerable. The main adverse effects reported with pioglitazone are those common to the TZD class: weight gain, pedal edema, bone loss and precipitation of congestive heart failure in at-risk individuals, without any increase in cardiovascular diseases /all-cause mortality. Overall, the safety profile of pioglitazone is favorable and remains a useful option for the treatment of insulin resistant patients (P. Shah, S Mudallar. 2010).

For choice of using insulin-sensitizing agents, High Molecular Weight (HMW) adiponectin is secreted from adipocytes and acts on increasing insulin sensitivity in target organs (T. Kadowaki, et al. 2005). HMW adiponectin is measured in sixty nine cases with non-PCOS and we determine normal range to be over 3.5μg/ml. Ovulation induction in PCOS is performed based on the property of metformin, pioglitazone and levels of adiponectin. In anovulatory PCOS subjects, GTT is first carried out. For positive insulin resistance (IR) with obesity, metformin (500~750mg) is chosen. When HMW adiponectin levels are in normal range for non-obese patients tested positive for IR, a 500mg dose of metformin is chosen, while a 7.5-15mg dose of Pioglitazone is chosen for those with low levels of HMW. For individuals with negative IR, HMW is measured so as to appropriately select either metformin or pioglitazone. Subjects with negative IR have to be abnormal in secretion patterns of insulin and / or glucose metabolic pattern by GTT. For the same subjects with normal levels of HMW adiponectin, metformin (250mg) is used while pioglitazone (7.5mg) is selected for low levels of HMW adiponectin. If ovulation induction with metformin or pioglitazone is failed during three to four cycles, clomiphen citrate is utilized along with one of the insulin sensitizing agents. It is also significant that improving life-style such as daily exercise and diet is highly recommended along with treatment using insulin sensitizing agents.

Ovulation induction in PCOS subjects is applied to 38 cases shown in Table 2. Ovulation rate is very high, 97.3 % (37/38). High pregnancy rate is also observed, 73.0% (27/37). Rate of combination use with clomiphen citrate is 36.8% (14/38). Therefore, the proposed management protocol satisfies treatment of patients with anovulatory PCOS.

Ovulation rate:	97.3% (37 / 38)	
Pregnancy rate:	73.0% (27 / 37)	
Abortion rate:	11.1% (3 / 27)	
Pregnancy rate with metformin:		69.2% (18 / 26)
Pregnancy rate with pioglitazone:		81.8% (9 / 11)
Rate of combination use with clomiphene citrate:		38.8% (14 / 38)

Table 2. Results of ovulation induction in PCOS subjects based on the properties of insulin sensitizing agents and levels of high molecular weight adiponectin.

7. Insulin resistance / hyperinsulinemia and implantation disorder

To study how insulin resistance / hyperinsulinemia affects implantation, GTT is carried out in seventy-eight subjects who failed implantation by the treatment of freeze-thawing embryo transfer method. Although embryos with good quality are transferred at least more than one time, pregnancy is not achieved. In this study, good quality embryos are defined as over four cells and less than 30% of fragmentation. Thirty five out of 78 cases reveal insulin resistance and / or hyperinsulinemia by GTT. Then, 11 out of 35 cases have PCOS. After treated with metformin, twenty out of 35 cases become pregnant by freeze-thawing embryo transfer. Six cases with PCOS become pregnant; five cases delivered and 1 case aborted. The results of this treatment are summarized in Table 3. The result indicates the possible ground implantation mechanisms.

Insulin resistance / hyperinsulinemia		35	cases
	(PCOS case)	(11	cases)
Pregnancy after treatment		20	cases
	(PCOS case)	(16	cases)
Delivered		16	cases
	(PCOS case)	(5	cases)
Aborted		4	cases
	(PCOS case)	(1	case)

Table 3. Results of implantation outcomes by freeze-thawing embryo transfer after treatment by insulin sensitizing agent (metformin).

According to Jakubowicz et al., glycodelin, insulin-like-growth factor-binding protein 1 (IGF-BP1), uterine vascularity and blood flow are studied for association with treatment of metformin and placebo in PCOS (DJ. Jakubowicz, et al. 2001). Glycodelin is a protein synthesized by secretary / decidualized endometrial glands. Circulating glycodelin may reflect endometrial function such as endometrial maturation and inhibition of endometrial immune response to the embryo (M. Seppala, et al. 1988; M. Julkunen, et al. 1990; AE. Bolton, et al. 1987; M. Julkunen, 1986; N. Okamoto, et al. 1991). IGF-BP1 is a protein that appears to facilitate adhesion process at the feto-maternal interface and may play an important role in the periimplantation period (LC. Giudice, et al. 1998; JI. Jones, et al. 1993). In comparison with placebo, metformin treatment increases concentration of glycodelin and

IGF-BP1 in luteal phase up to 3 to 4-fold. Besides, it increases in vascular penetration and increase in blood flow of spiral arteries that is demonstrated by 20% reduction in the resistance index. From this, endometrial function and amelioration of its environment may be improved by treatment of hyperinsulinemia, which has a strong correlation with insulin resistance and PCOS.

8. Insulin resistance / hyperinsulinemia and early pregnancy loss

Women with PCOS are associated with 30 - 50% of early pregnancy loss at a higher risk than normal women (L. Regan, et al. 1990; HR. Gray, et al. 2000). They are also involved in 36 - 82% of the risk for recurrent early pregnancy loss (HS. Liddell, et al. 1997). Treatment of insulin sensitizing agents is applied to 38 cases with PCOS that resulted in ovulation of 37 cases. As shown in Table 3, twenty seven cases became pregnant after the treatment. Then, the abortion rate is 11.1% (three out of 27 cases) that is almost as low as that of normal women. This explains treatment of insulin sensitizing agents might be effective for sustaining early pregnancy periods. This concept can be also emphasized (DJ. Jackbowicz, et al. 2002), the rate of early pregnancy loss is 8.8% as compared with 41.9% for control group in PCOS. Metformin therapy during pregnancy in women with PCOS is safely associated with reduction of spontaneous abortion for the first trimester and is not teratogenic without adverse effects on biological and physical conditions of baby. In addition, metformin therapy improves the insulin level, HOMA- R and high plasminogen activator inhibitor activity (PAI-Fx) (CJ. Glueck, et al. 2002). Therefore, metformin therapy that has insulin-lowering effect might be accountable for protecting early pregnancy loss. Nevertheless, sustaining the pregnancy might be achieved through lifestyle intervention.

9. Conclusion

PCOS is a very common complex that occurs in approximately up to 20% of women of reproductive age and threatens fertility and metabolic condition as well. And also, it is chronic diseases, such as dyslipidemia, type 2 diabetes and cardiovascular diseases, across the lifespan. These conditions represent a major health and financial burden. It is mentioned that PCOS is the beginning of lifestyle-related diseases. Although it is still challenging to fully comprehend and reveal this unknown syndrome for researchers, PCOS has been known to be involved in insulin resistance / hyperinsulinemia. It is well-known that insulin resistance / hyperinsulinemia is affected by lifestyle factors, such as diet and physical activities. As mentioned above, approximately 5 to 10% of weight loss is enough to ameliorate ovulatory dysfunction and metabolic disorders. Therefore, the improvement of lifestyle is a key to overcoming reproductive and metabolic disorders in women with PCOS. Also, the efficacy of insulin sensitizing agents may contribute to the amelioration of insulin resistance / hyperinsulinemia and be also effective for the reproductive and metabolic functions of PCOS women. Insulin sensitizing agents consequently facilitate ovulation, implantation and maintenance of pregnancy. As reiterated, both lifestyle management and appropriate medication might be conductive to the improvement of adverse effects for reproductive processes by insulin resistance / hyperinsulinemia in PCOS (S. Franks. 2011; T. Sakumoto, et al. 2010). Nevertheless, it requires further study for comprehension of PCOS. More understanding of the complexity of PCOS might lead to optimal management of PCOS for clinicians and patients.

The relationship between differentiation of visceral adipocytes and reproductive processes is shown in Fig 2 (T. Yamauchi, et al. 2001; T. Sakumoto, et al. 2010).

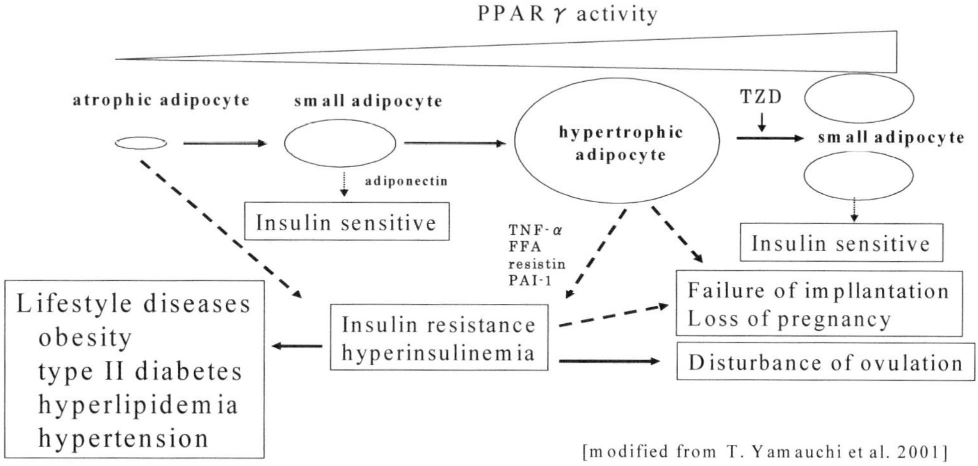

FFA : free fatty acid, PAI-1 : plasminogen activator inhibitor 1,
PPAR-γ: peroxisome proliferator-activated receptor gamma
TNF-α: tumor necrosis factor alpha, TZD: thiazolidinedione

Fig. 2. The relationship between differentiation of visceral adipocytes and reproductive processes (T. Sakumoto, et al. 2010)

10. Acknowledgement

We would like to express gratitude to Ms. Eun-Ju Choi for proofreading of the manuscript.

11. References

Abdul-Ghani, MA. Jenkinson, CP. Richardson, DK. Tripathy, D. DeFronzo, RA. (2006a). Insulin secretion and action in subjects with impaired fasting glucose and impaired glucose tolerance: Results from the veterans administration genetic epidemiology study. *Diabetes*. 55, 1430–1435.

Acien, P. Quereda, F. Matalin, P. Vilarroya, E. Lopez-Fernandez, JA. Acien, M. Mauri, Monserrat, Alfayatte, R. (1999). Insulin, androgens, and obesity in women with and without polycystic ovary syndrome: A heterogeneous group of disorders. *Fertil Steril*. 72 32-40.

Ahre´n, B. Larsson, H. (2002). Quantification of insulin secretion in relation to insulin sensitivity in nondiabetic postomenopausal women. *Diabetes*. 52:202-211.

Alibegovic, AC. Højbjerre, L. Sonne, MP. van Hall, G. Stallknecht, B. Dela, F. Vaag, A. (2009). Impact of nine days of bed rest on hepatic and peripheral insulin action, insulin secretion and whole body lipolysis in healthy young male offspring of patients with type 2 diabetes. *Diabetes*. 58, 2749–2756.

Attia GR, Rainey WE, Carr BR. (2001). Metformin directly inhibits androgen production in human thecal cells. *Fertil Steril*. 76: 517-24

Barbien, RL. Smith, S. Ryun, KJ. (1988). The role of hyperinsulinemia in the pathogenesis of ovarian hyperandrogenism. *Fertil Steril.* 50: 197-212

Barbieri, RL. Makris, A. Randall, RW. (1986). Insulin stimulates androgen accumulation on incubation of ovarian stroma obtained from women with hyperandrogenism. *J Clin Endocrinol Metab.* 62: 904-10

Baysal, B. Batukun, M. Batukun, C. (2001). Biochemical and body weight changes with metformin in polycystic ovary syndrome. *Clin Exp Obsetet Gynecol.* 28:212-4.

Bolton AE, Pockley AG, Clough KJ, Mowles EA, Stoker RJ, Westwood OM, Chapman MG. (1987). Identification of placental protein 14 as an immunosuppressive factor in human reproduction. *Lancet.* 1: 593-5

Botwood, N. Hamilton-Fairly, D. Kiddy, D. (1995). Sex hormone-binding globulin and female reproductive function. *J Steroid Biochem Mol Biol.* 53: 529-31

Brøns, C. Jensen, CB. Storgaard, H. Hiscock, NJ. White, A, Appel, JS. Jacobsen, S. Nilsson, E.

Carmina, E. Koyama, T. Chang, L. Stanczyk, FZ. Lobo, RA. (1992). Does ethnicity influence the prevalence of adrenal hyperandrogenism and insulin resistance in polycystic ovary syndrome?. *Am J Obstet Gynecol.* 167: 1807-12

Chang, RJ. Nakamura, RM. Judd, HL. Kaplan, SA. (1983). Insulin resistance in nonobese patients with polycystic ovarian disease. *J Clin Endocrinol Metab.* 57: 356-9

Cobelli C, Toffolo GM, Man CD, Campioni M, Denti P, Caumo A, Butler P, Rizza R. (2007). Assessment of β-cell function in humans, simultaneously with insulin sensitivity and hepatic extraction, from intravenous and oral glucose tests. *Am J Physiol Endocrinol Metab.* 293:E1-15.

Dunaif, A. Ginf, M. Mandeli, J. Laumas, V. Dobrjansky, A. (1987). Characterization of groups of hyperandrogenemic women with acanthosis nigricans, impaired glucose tolerance, and/or hyperinsulinemia . *J Clin Endocrinol Metab.* 65: 499-507

Dunaif, A. Segal, KR. Futterweil, W. Dobrjansky, A. (1989). Profound peripheral insulin resistance independent of obesity in polycystic syndrome. Diabetes. 38: 1165-74

Dunaif, A. Segal, KR. Shelley, DR. Green, G. Dobrjansky, A. Licholan, T. (1992). Evidence for distinctive and intrinsic defects in insulin action in polycystic ovary syndrome. *Diabetes.* 41: 1257-66

Ehrmann, DA. Rosenfield, RL. Barnes, RB. Brigell, DF. Sheikh, Z. (1992). Detection of functional ovarian hyperandrogenism in women with androgen excess. *N Engl J Med.* 327: 157-62

Ehrmann, DA. Sturis, J. Byrne, MM. Karrison, T. Rosenfield, RL. Polonsky, KS. (1995). Insulin secretory defects in polycystic ovary syndrome. Relationship to insulin sensitivity and family history of non-insulin-dependent diabetes mellitus. *J Clin Invest.* 96: 520-27

Færch, K. Brøns. C, Alibegovic, A.C. Vaag, A. (2010). The disposition index: adjustment for peripheral vs. hepatic insulin sensitivity? *J Physiol.* 588.5:59-764.

Færch, K. Vaag, A. Holst, J. Glumer, C. Pedersen, O. Borch-Johnsen, K. (2008). Impaired fasting glycaemia vs impaired glucose tolerance: similar impairment of pancreatic alpha and beta cell function but differential roles of incretin hormones and insulin action. *Diabetologia* 51, 853–861.

Farrell, K. Antoni, MH. (2010). Insulin resistance, obesity, inflammation, and depression in polycystic ovary syndrome: biobehavioral mechanisms and interventions. *Fertil Steril.* 94:1565-1574.

Fauser, BCJM. (2003). The Rotterdam ESHRE/ASRM-Sponsored PCOS consensus workshop group: Revised 2003 consensus on diagnostic criteria and long-term health risks related to polycystic ovary syndrome (PCOS). *Hum Reprod* 19:41-47.

Fleming, R. Hopkinson, ZE. Wallance, AM. Greer, IA. Greer, IA. Sattar, N. (2002). Ovarian function and metabolic factors in women with oligomenorrhea treated with metformin in randomized double blind placebo-controlled trail. *J Clin Endocrinol Metab.* 87:569-74.

Fornes, R. Ormazabal, P. Rosas, C. Gabler, F. Vantman, D. Romero, C. Vega, M. (2010). Changes in the expression of insulin signaling pathway molecules in endometria from plycystic ovary syndrome women with or without hypderinsulinemia. *Mol Med.* 16:129-136.

Franks S, Gilling-Smith C, Waston H, Willis D. (1999). Insulin action in the normal and polycystic ovary. *Endocrinol Metab Clin N Am.* 28: 361-78

Franks S, Robinson S, Willis D. (1996). Nutrition, insulin and polycystic ovary syndrome. *Reviews of Reproduction.* 1: 47-53.

Franks, S. (2011). When should an insulin sensitizing agent be used in the treatment of polycystic ovary syndrome? *Clinical endocrinology.* 74:148-151.

Freeman, R. Pollack, R. Rosenbloom, E. (2010). Assessing impaired glucose tolerance and insulin resistance in Polycystic Ovarian Syndrome with a muffin test: Alternative to glucose tolerance test. *Endocr Pract.* 1-24.

Fulghesu, A. Magnini, R. Portoghese, E. Angioni, S. Minerba, L. Melis, GB. (2011) Obesity-related lipid profile and altered insulin incretion in adolescents with polycystic ovary syndrome. *J Adolesc Health.* 474-481

Galletly, C. Clark, A. Tomlinson, L. Blaney, F. (1996). A group program for obese, infertile women: weight loss and improved psychological health. *J Psychosom Obstet Gynaecol.* 17:125-128.

Giudice LC, Mark SP, Irwin JC. (1998). Paracrine actions of insulin-like growth factors and IGF binding protein-1 in non-pregnant human endometrium and at the decidual-trophoblast interface. *J Reprod Immunol.* 39: 133-48

Glueck CJ, Wang P, Goldenberg N, Sieve-Smith L. (2002). Pregnancy outcomes among women with polycystic ovary syndrome treated with metformin. *Hum Reprod.* 17: 2858-64

Gray HR, Wu LY. (2000). Subfertility and risk of spontaneous abortion. *Am J Public Health.* 90: 1452-54

Hillier SG. (1994). Current concepts of the roles of follicle stimulating hormone and luteinizing hormone in folliculogenesis. *Hum Reprod.* 9: 188-91

Jakubowicz DJ, Iuorno MJ, Jakubowicz S, Roberts KA, Nestler JE. (2002). Effects of metformin on early pregnancy loss in the polycystic ovary syndrome. *J Clin Endocrinol Metab.* 87: 524-29

Jakubowicz DJ,Seppala M, Jakubowicz S, Rodriguez-Arms O, Rivas-Santiago A, Koistinen H, Koistine R, Nestler JE. (2001). Insulin reduction with metformin increases luteal phase serum glycodelin and insulin-like growth factor-binding protein 1 concentrations and enhances uterine vascularity and blood flow in the polycystic ovary syndrome. *J Clin Endocrinol Metab.* 86: 1126-33

Jones JI, Gockerman A, Busby WHJ, Wright G, Glemmons DR. (1993). Insulin-like growth factor binding protein 1 stimulates cell migration and binds to the α5β1 integrin by means of its Arg-Gly-Asp sequence. *Proc Natl Acad Sci USA*. 90: 10553-7

Julkunen M, Koistinen R, Suikkari AM, Seppala M, Janne OA. (1990). Identification by hybridization histochemistry of human endometrial cells expressing mRNAs encoding a uterine β-lactogloblin homologue and insulin-like growth factor-binding protein-1. *Mol Endocrinol*. 4: 700-7

Julkunen M, Koiteinen R, Sjoberg J, Rutanen EM, Wahlstrom T, Seppala M. (1986). Secretary endometrium synthesizes placental protein 14. *Endocrinolgy*. 118: 1782-6

Kadowaki T and Yamauchi T. (2005). Adiponectin and adiponectin receptors. *Endocrine Reviews*. 26: 439-51

Laakso, M. Zilinskaite ,J. Hansen, T. Boesgaard, T. Vanttinen, M. Stanc´akov´a, A. Jansson, PA. Pellm´e, F. Holst, J. Kuulasmaa, T. Hribal, M. Sesti, G. Stefan, N. Fritsche, A. Haring, H. Pedersen, O. Smith, U. for the EUGENE2 Consortium. (2008). Insulin sensitivity, insulin release and glucagon-like peptide-1 levels in persons with impaired fasting glucose and/or impaired glucose tolerance in the EUGENE 2 study. *Diabetologia* 51:502-511.

Larsen, CM. Astrup, A. Quistorff, B. Vaag, A. (2009). Impact of short-term high-fat feeding on glucose and insulin metabolism in young healthy men. *J Physiol*. 587, 2387–2397.

Liddell HS, Sowden K, Farquhar CM. (1997). Reccurent miscarriage: screening for polycystic ovaries and subsequent pregnancy outcome. *Aust NZJ Obstet Gynaecol*. 37: 402-6

Lim, SS. Norman, RJ. Glifton, PM. Noakes, M. (2009). Hyperandrogenemia, psychological distress, and food cravings in young women. *Physiol Behav*. 98(3):276-80.

Matthews DR, Hosker JP, Rudenski AS, Naylor BA, Treacher DF, Turner RC. (1985). Homeostasis model assessment: insulin resistance and beta-cell function from fasting plasma glucose and insulin concentrations in man. *Diabetologia*. 28: 412-19

Mcyer F, Ipaktchi M, Clauser H. (1967). Specific inhibition of gluconeogenesis by biguanides . *Nature*. 213: 203-4

Moran, LJ. Hutchison, SK. Norman, RJ. Teede, HJ. (2011). Lifestyle changes in women with polycystic ovary syndrome. *Cochrane Database Syst Rev*. Issue 2.

Moran, LJ. Pasquali, R. Teede, HJ. Hoeger, KM. Norman, RJ. (2009). Treatment of obesity in polycystic ovary syndrome: a position statement of the Androgen Excess and Polycystic Ovary Syndrome Society. *Fertil Steril*. 92(6):1966-82.

Murray, RD. Davison, RM. Russell, RC. (2000). Clinical presentation of PCOS following development of an insulinoma. Case report. Hum Reprod. 15: 86-8

Nahum, R. Thong, KJ. Hillier, SG. (1995). Metabolic regulation of androgen production by human theca cells in vitro. *Hum Reprod*. 10: 75-81

Nestler, JE. Stovall, D. Akhter, N. Juorno, MJ. Jakubowics, DJ. (2002). Strategies for the use of insulin-sensitizing drugs to treat infertility in women with polycystic ovary syndrome. *Fertile Steril*. 77:209-15.

Norman, RJ. Davies, MJ. Lord, J. Moran, LJ. (2002). The role of lifestyle modification in polycystic ovary syndrome. *Trends Endocrinol Metab*. 13:251-7.

Okamoto N, Uchida A, Takakura K, Karuya Y, Kanzaki H, Riittinen L, Koistinene R, Seppala M, Mori T. (1991). Suppression by human placental protein 14 of natural killer cell activity. *Am J Reprod Immunol*. 26: 137-42

Ovalle, F. Azziz, R. (2002). Insulin resistance, polycystic ovary syndrome, and type 2 diabetes mellitus. *Fertil Steril.* 77:1095-1105.

Pesant, MH. Baillargeon, JP. (2011). Clinically useful predictors of conversion to abnormal glucose tolerance in women with polycystic ovary syndrome. *Fertil Steril.* 95:210-215.

Poehlman, ET. Dvorak, RV. DeNino, WF. Brochu, M. Ades, PA. (2000). Effects of resistance training and endurance training on insulin sensitivity in nonobese, young women: a controlled randomized trial. *J Clin Endocrinol Metab.* 85:2463-2468.

Regan L, Owen EJ, Jacobs HS. (1990). Hypersecretion of luteinising hormone, infertility, and miscarriage. *Lancet.* 336: 1141-44

Rosenfield, RL.Barnes, RB. Cara, JF. Licky, AW. (1990). Dysregulation of cytochrome P450c17 alpha as the cause of polycystic ovarian syndrome. *Fertil Steril.* 53: 785-91

Sakumoto, T. Tokunaga, Y. Tanaka, H. Nohara, M. Motegi, E. Shinkawa, T. Nakaza, A. Higashi, M. (2010). Insulin resistance / hyperinsulinemia and reproductive disorders in infertile women. *Reprod Med Biol.* 9:185-190.

Seppala M, Riittinen L, Julkunen M, Koistinen R, Wahlstrom T, Iino K, Alfthan H, Stenman UH, Huhtala ML. (1988). Structural studies, localization in tissue and clinical aspect of human endometrial proteins. *J Reprod Fertil Suppl.* 36: 127-41

Shah P, Muddaliar S. (2010). Pioglitazone: side effect and safety profile. *Expert Opin Drug Saf.* 9:347-54.

Strowitzki, T. Capp, E. von Eye Corleta, H. (2010). The degree of cycle irregularity correlates with the grade of endocrine and metabolic disorders in PCOS patients. *Eur J Obstet Gynecol Reprod Biol.* 149:178-181.

Suikkan, AM. Koivisto, VA. Korstinen, R. (1989). Dose-response characteristics for suppression of low molecular weight plsma insulin-like growth factor-binding protein by insulin. *J Clin Endocrinol Metab.* 68:135-40

Suikkan, AM. Koivisto, VA. Rutanen, EM. (1988). Insulin regulates the serum levels of low molecular weight insulin-like growth factor-binding protein. *J Clin Endocrinol Metab.* 66: 266-72

Takikawa, S. Iwase, A. Goto, M. Harata, T. Umezu, T. Nakahara, T. Kobayashi, H. Suzuki, K. Manabe, S. Kikkawa, F. (2010). Assessment of the predictive value of follicular fulid insulin, leptin and adiponectin in assisted reproductive cycles. *Gynecol Endocrinol.* 26:494-499.

Tanaka H, Shimabukuro T, Shimabukuro M. (2005). High prevalence of metabolic syndrome among men in Okinawa. *J Atheroscler Thromb.* 12:284-8.

Traub, ML. (2011). Assessing and treating insulin resistance in women with polycystic ovarian syndrome. *World J Diabetes.* 2: 33-40.

Vrbikova, J. Hill, M. Starka, L. Vondra, K. (2002). Predication of the effect of metformin treatment in patients with polycystic ovary syndrome. Gynecol Obstet Invest. 53:100-4.

Wang, JX. Davies, MJ. Norman, RJ. (2002). Obesity increases the risk of spontaneous abortion during infertility treatment. *Obes Res.* 10:551-4.

Willis, DS. Watson, H. Mason, HD. Galea, R. Brincat, M. Franks, S. (1998). Premature response to luteinizing hormone of granulosa cells from anovulatory women with polycystic ovary syndrome relevance to mechanism anovulation. *J Clin Endocrinol Metab.* 83: 3984-91

Wollen N, Bailey CJ. (1988). Inhibition of hepatic gluconeogenesis by metformin. Synergism with insulin. *Biochem Pharmacol*. 37; 4353-8

Yamauchi T, Kamon J, Waki H, Murakami K, Motojima K,Komeda K, Ide T, Kubota N, Terauchi Y, Tobe K, Miki H, Tsuchida A, Akanuma Y, Nagai R, Kimura S, Kadowaki T. (2001). The mechanisms by which both heterozygous peroxisome proliferator-activated receptorγ (PPARγ) deficiency and PPARγ agonist improve insulin resistance. *J Biol Chem*. 276: 41245-54